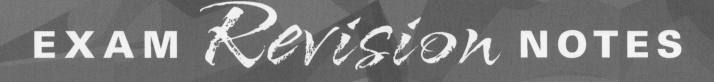

EXAM *Revision* NOTES

AS/A-LEVEL

PE/Sport Studies

2nd Edition

Carl Atherton
Symond Burrows
Sue Young

Philip Allan Updates, an imprint of Hodder Education, part of Hachette Livre UK, Market Place, Deddington, Oxfordshire OX15 0SE

Orders

Bookpoint Ltd, 130 Milton Park, Abingdon, Oxfordshire OX14 4SB
tel: 01235 827720
fax: 01235 400454
e-mail: uk.orders@bookpoint.co.uk

Lines are open 9.00 a.m.–5.00 p.m., Monday to Saturday, with a 24-hour message answering service. You can also order through the Philip Allan Updates website: www.philipallan.co.uk

© Philip Allan Updates 2008

ISBN 978-0-340-95858-2

First printed 2008

Impression number	5	4	3	2	1
Year	2012	2011	2010	2009	2008

Printed in Spain

Hachette Livre UK's policy is to use papers that are natural, renewable and recyclable products and made from wood grown in sustainable forests. The logging and manufacturing processes are expected to conform to the environmental regulations of the country of origin

P01246

Contents

Introduction

About this book

This book is a concise summary of the elements you need to know to help you prepare your revision for AS/A-level PE. It includes essential information needed to answer questions on the main topics covered by the PE specifications of the main exam boards.

The book is divided into three sections. The first section concentrates on anatomy and physiology, the second section focuses on skills acquisition and sports psychology, and the third section covers social and historical studies. Each section is further divided into a number of topics.

How to use these notes

Use this book in conjunction with your own notes and the specification from your particular exam board. The exam boards differ slightly in the detail they require and, within some topics, in the actual content covered.

Try to start your revision early so that you do not have to do too much at once. One or two topics from this guide are enough for one session. At the start of each topic, there is a checklist of the information you need to know before you go into the exam room. Use this list to monitor your knowledge as you work your way through the material. By setting a goal for each session and ticking off your progress, your confidence will grow. Once you have read the main core of each topic, you could condense the information onto flash cards including just the key words; these cards will serve to prompt your memory into recalling the more detailed content you have read. Carry these cards around with you to test yourself. Throughout this guide, the key words are often given in bold type.

Each topic contains examiner tips, which give advice on the points that create most problems for students. They also highlight where there are differences between the exam boards in terms of content. Take careful note of these tips and make sure that you remember them in your revision as well as the exam.

Revising for AS and A-level PE

The only way to ensure success in the exam is to make sure you revise thoroughly. By knowing your subject matter, you will recognise the requirements of the questions and be more confident of answering correctly.

Revision is personal. Some students like to read and re-read, others would rather make notes; some like to work with a partner or group of friends and others prefer to be alone and quiet. The best advice is to do what suits *you*. Whichever method you choose, the following guidelines will be useful.

Make a plan
You should complete a revision plan as early as possible, using the checklists contained in these notes and your exam specification. Start your plan with the topics you find the most difficult, so that you can get help and revisit these later if necessary. Make a revision timetable and stick to it. Allow yourself regular breaks and some leisure time

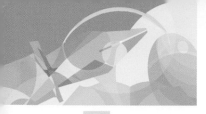

— if you start your revision early enough, you will have time for relaxation, such as a night out or a visit to the gym. Those who start revising too late go into the exam tired, full of last-minute panic and unable to do themselves justice. In some cases, you may be studying 4 or even 5 subjects, and you will probably need 4 weeks to complete your revision for each module of study within those subjects. Allow some flexibility within your timetable so that you can cope with any sudden unexpected events, such as a late invitation to a party or a family crisis.

Do quality revision

When revising, it is what you do that counts, not how long you do it for. In each revision session, concentrate on the task in hand and focus on one topic. Have a break after an hour or so and then return to it. If you reach a point when you feel you are no longer taking anything in, allow yourself a break, have a coffee, and relax for a short while, rather than let frustration get the better of you. Once you are focused again, you can return to your revision in a calmer state of mind.

Set goals

Use the checklists in this book and your own notes to set a target that you want to reach in each revision session. Be prepared to adjust these targets if you are finding them too difficult or too easy. Once you are confident you have reached a target, tick it off on your checklist.

Practise skills and techniques

While you may have the knowledge, you still need to be able to put it into practice. Make sure that you can answer questions using the factual knowledge you have gained. Ask for copies of past papers, and test yourself or ask someone else to test you. Most importantly, get to know how the examiners work so that you can understand the principles behind each question and what the examiner is looking for.

Start early

Don't put off your revision. Begin your focused reading and note taking as early as possible, in order to build up knowledge and understanding of your PE course in a steady and progressive way.

Exam technique

The factual knowledge you bring to the exam is only worthwhile if you can present it to the examiner in the correct format. Quite often, hard work during the course and solid revision is wasted because students show poor technique in the exam. The basic steps to good exam technique are summarised in the chart below. Keep this process in mind as you answer each question and use it to check your response at the end of the exam.

Planning your answer — what should I include?

↓

Key points — have I made enough points to gain full marks?

↓

Verbs — what is the examiner asking me to do?

↓

Examples — can I think of any to illustrate my answer?

Planning your answer

Spend a few minutes thinking about and preparing your answer, and focus carefully on the question before you start to write. This will make sure that your answer is presented neatly, as there will be less chance of errors and subsequent crossings out.

Write a brief plan before you begin your full answer for questions that are relatively high in their mark allocations (i.e 4 or more marks), to ensure that you do not miss anything out. Read and re-read the question and highlight the key words, referring back to these as you write up your answer. The time spent planning will be worth it.

When you write your answer, do so in an examiner-friendly way, so that there are spaces between each part. Remember that some of the points you make could be written as a bulleted list so that they stand out and can be identified clearly. Write your answers in the order the questions appear on the exam paper and do not leave any gaps — if you do not know the answer, make an educated guess.

Key points

One of the biggest failings in students' answers is that they simply do not say enough. The examiner has a mark scheme listing a number of key points or phrases for which the candidate can be awarded a mark. If you hit the key point, you get the mark. Quite often the question will give you a strong hint by putting a phrase in italics.

If the question is worth 5 marks, there may be 7 or 8 key points for which you can get credit. Marks are not deducted for a wrong answer, so cover yourself and give more answers than there are marks available. Therefore, write at least 7 answers for a 5-mark question.

Verbs

These are action words — the task the examiner is asking you to do — so make sure you respond in the appropriate way. The following are some of the main tasks you are required to perform in an A-level PE exam:

- **Compare:** identify similarities and differences between particular topics.
- **Define:** give a precise meaning of a term.
- **Describe:** give an account of the main features.
- **Explain:** give causes/reasons. You need to check your answer to this question by asking yourself, have I said *why*? This takes a description one step further.
- **Name, identify or list:** a series of one-word answers or short phrases might be sufficient here. You do not need to rewrite the question in your response, but you might introduce your one-word answers with a simple sentence. For example, in response to the question 'name three characteristics of skilful movement in sport', you might say: 'Three characteristics of skilful movement are:
  – evidence of learning
  – aesthetic quality
  – consistency'
- **Sketch:** draw a simple diagram or illustrate a graph without having to show exact figures.
- **State:** a short, concise answer is needed here. Again, the key points will get the marks.

Section 1
Anatomy & physiology

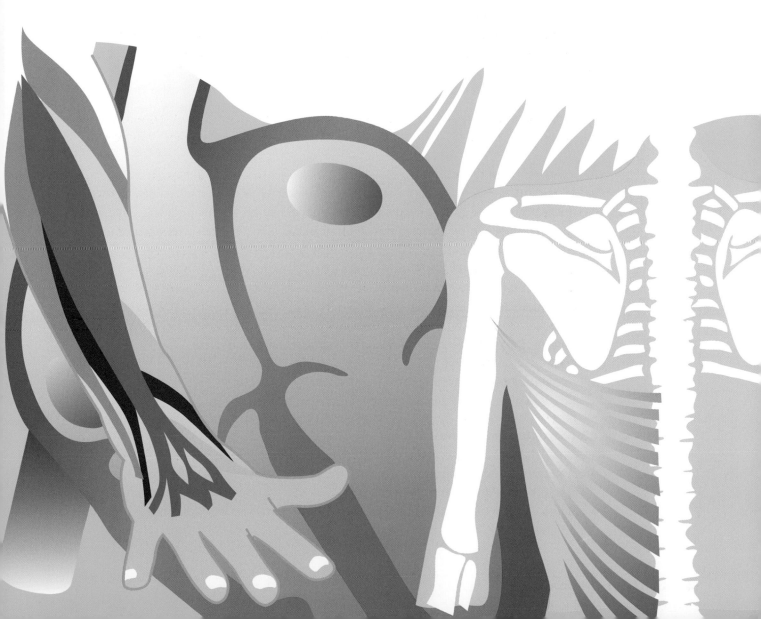

Movement analysis

By the end of this topic, you should be able to:

- classify the different types of joint in the body according to how much movement they allow
- identify the bones particular to each joint type
- list the different types of muscular contraction and the functions of different muscles
- explain how joints, movement and muscles are connected, and give examples
- evaluate the impact of different types of physical activity on both the skeletal and muscular systems

1 Joints

The skeleton is a framework of bones connected by joints. Joints are necessary for muscles to lever bones and create movement, and are formed where any two or more bones meet. There are three types of joint, classified by how much movement they allow: **fibrous**, **cartilaginous** and **synovial**.

1.1 Fibrous joint

A fibrous joint allows no movement at all; it is completely fixed. There is no joint cavity and the bones are held together by fibrous, connective tissue. Examples of this type of joint can be found in the cranium, facial bones and pelvic girdle.

1.2 Cartilaginous joint

A cartilaginous joint allows only a slight amount of movement, as the bones are separated by cartilage. Examples of this type of joint are the ribs joining the sternum and the vertebrae joining to form the spine.

1.3 Synovial joint

Synovial joints are the most common type of joint and allow movement in one or more directions. They have a fluid-filled cavity surrounded by an articular capsule. Hyaline/articular cartilage can be found where the bones come into contact with each other.

1.3a Types of synovial joint

There are six types of synovial joint:

- **ball and socket** joint (e.g. hip and shoulder)
- **hinge** joint (e.g. ankle, knee and elbow)
- **pivot** joint (e.g. between the axis and atlas vertebrae in the neck)
- **saddle** joint (e.g. thumb)
- **condyloid** joint (e.g. wrist)
- **gliding** joint (e.g. between adjacent vertebrae in the spine)

1.3b Structure of a synovial joint

All synovial joints have several common features. These include:

- **articular/hyaline cartilage**, which covers the ends of the bones at a joint and prevents friction between the articulating bones
- a **joint capsule** — a tough, fibrous layer of tissue encasing the joint, which protects and strengthens it

- a **synovial membrane** — the inner layer or lining of the joint capsule, which secretes synovial fluid
- **synovial fluid**, which fills the joint capsule, nourishing the articular cartilage and preventing friction
- **ligament** — strong, fibrous connective tissue that provides stability by joining bone to bone
- **pads of fat**, which act as shock absorbers in the joint
- **bursae** — fluid-filled sacs located between the tendon and a bone that reduce friction and wear and tear

2   *Movement terminology*

- **abduction:** movement occurring away from the midline of the body
- **adduction:** movement occurring towards the midline of the body
- **circumduction:** through a combination of flexion, extension, abduction and adduction, the lower end of the bone moves around in a circle
- **depression:** moving the shoulders downwards
- **dorsiflexion:** bending the foot upwards towards the tibia/bending the hand backwards
- **elevation:** moving the shoulders upwards (remember that this movement occurs from the shoulder girdle)
- **extension:** an increase in the angle that occurs around a joint
- **flexion:** a decrease in the angle that occurs around a joint
- **horizontal extension** (also called horizontal abduction): moving the arm backward across the body at 90 degrees to shoulder abduction
- **horizontal flexion** (also called horizontal adduction): moving the arm forward across the body at 90 degrees to shoulder abduction
- **lateral flexion:** bending sideways
- **palmar flexion:** bending the hand downwards towards the inside of the forearm
- **plantar flexion:** bending the foot downwards away from the tibia (standing on tiptoes)
- **pronation:** facing the palm of the hand downwards
- **rotation:** movement of a bone around its axis; this rotation can be inward (medial) or outward (lateral)
- **supination:** facing the palm of the hand upwards (carrying a 'soup' bowl may help you to remember)

3   *Types of muscular contraction*

A muscle can contract in three different ways — **concentric**, **eccentric** or **isometric** — depending on the muscle action that is required.

3.1 Concentric contraction

This is when a muscle shortens under tension. For example, during the upward phase of an arm curl, the biceps brachii perform a concentric contraction as they shorten to produce flexion of the elbow.

3.2 Eccentric contraction

This is when the muscle lengthens under tension and does not relax. When a muscle contracts eccentrically, it is acting as a brake in helping to control movement during negative work. An example is landing from a standing jump. Here, the quadriceps are performing negative work as they are supporting the weight of the body during landing. The knee joint is in the flexed position but the quadriceps are unable to relax, as the weight of the body ensures that they lengthen under tension.

All muscle action is controlled by internal regulatory mechanisms such as **proprioceptors** (sense organs that provide feedback of the body's movement), **muscle spindle apparatus** (sensitive receptors between muscle fibres that relay information about the state of muscle contraction and the muscle's degree of stretch) and **golgi tendon organs** (which trigger a reflex action when a high tension develops in a muscle, causing it to shorten).

4 Muscle function

A muscle can perform four functions:

(1) When a muscle shortens under tension to produce movement it is an **agonist**.

(2) When a muscle returns to its original length it acts as an **antagonist**.

(3) A **fixator** muscle increases in tension but no movement occurs. It is normally located at the joint where the origin of the agonist can be found. In the upward phase of an arm curl, for example, the biceps brachia contracts and is the agonist. Its origin can be found on the shoulder, so the deltoid acts as a fixator during this movement.

(4) **Synergist** refers to a muscle that assists the work of an agonist.

5 Joints, movement and muscles

Synovial joint	Example	Bones that articulate movement	Movements	Agonist (muscle producing movement)
Ball and socket	Hip	Acetabulum of the pelvis and femur	Flexion Extension Outward rotation Inward rotation Abduction Adduction	Ilio psoas Gluteus maximus Gluteus maximus Gluteus minimus Gluteus maximus Adductors (longus, brevis and magnus)
	Shoulder	Glenoid fossa of the scapula and humerus	Flexion Extension Outward rotation Inward rotation Abduction Adduction Horizontal extension Horzontal flexion	Anterior deltoid Latissimus dorsi Infraspinatus Subscapularis Middle deltoid Pectoralis major Latissimus dorsi Pectoralis major

Synovial joint	Example	Bones that articulate movement	Movements	Agonist (muscle producing movement)
Hinge	Elbow	Radius, ulna and humerus	Flexion Extension	Biceps brachii Triceps brachii
	Knee	Tibia, femur and patella	Flexion Extension	Biceps femoris Rectus femoris
	Ankle	Tibia, fibula and talus	Plantar flexion Dorsiflexion	Gastrocnemius Tibialis anterior
Pivot	Neck	Atlas and axis	Rotation	
	Radio-ulna	Radius and ulna	Pronation Supination	Pronator teres Supinator
Gliding	Spine	Vertebral arches	Flexion Extension Lateral flexion Rotation (to the opposite side)	Rectus abdominus Sacrospinalis External obliques External obliques
Condyloid	Wrist	Carpals, radius, ulna	Palmar flexion Dorsiflexion	Wrist flexors Wrist extensors

Examiner's tip

Learning the data in the above table will give you all the necessary information, but make sure you can apply your knowledge. For AQA, you are asked to look at specific movements, so you only need to revise the ankle, knee, hip, shoulder and elbow.

6 Impact of exercise on the skeletal system

6.1 Low-impact aerobic activity

Low-impact aerobic activity can help to prevent **demineralisation**, a process whereby calcium salts are lost and a condition known as osteoporosis may develop (weakening of the bones). Bones become stronger as calcium deposits build up, and the strength of muscles, tendons and ligaments is likewise increased. This type of activity:

● avoids overuse injuries by varying the line of stress on bone
● can improve the symptoms of mild osteoarthritis by nourishing cartilage and bone and strengthening and stabilising the joints

6.2 Strength training/core stability

Strength training/core stability can cause **hypertrophy** of the muscles. This increase in muscle strength leads to an increase in joint stability. For example, core stability exercises will increase the strength of the rotator cuff muscles and increase stability in the shoulder joint, as well as reducing the likelihood of problems with the lumbar vertebrae. Increasing the strength in the quadriceps muscles will help stabilise tracking and knee function.

Strengthening exercises can also help with mild osteoarthritis by decreasing joint stiffness and strengthening the muscles around a joint to give protection and absorb shock. However, there are a lot of eccentric muscle contractions in strength training, which can cause muscle damage when pushed to maximum.

6.3 High-impact activities

High-impact activities involve contact, for example a tackle in rugby or a landing in the triple jump. Such activities can cause damage to **growth plates** — the softer parts of young people's bones where growth occurs. They are located at the end of a bone and are the weakest sections of the skeleton. Due to the fragile nature of growth plates, they are susceptible to injury. Immediate treatment is required in the event of injury, as it can affect how the bone grows.

Contact causing side impact on joints can occur in a slide tackle in football. This can cause medial or cruciate ligament damage in the knee. The shoulder joint has a shallow joint cavity, so high impact can cause dislocation.

6.4 Flexibility training

Flexibility training can increase the resting length of tendons, ligaments and muscles surrounding a joint due to greater elasticity, although there is a much bigger increase in muscle tissue. This will extend the range of movement around the joint. However, extreme flexibility can stretch ligaments, which in turn leads to a lack of stability.

6.5 Activities involving repetitive movements/overuse

Activities involving repetitive movements/overuse can place too much stress upon a part of the body, resulting in injury. This may manifest itself in:
- inflammation of the bursa
- wearing down of articular/hyaline cartilage in joints
- muscle strain or tissue damage

In children and teenagers, most overuse injuries occur at the growth plates. The most common repetitive stress injuries can be found at the elbows, shoulders, knees and heels.

6.6 Speed/agility training

Speed/agility training allows muscles to retain more elasticity/elastin, which means they can contract with more speed and power.

2 Mechanics, motion and movement

By the end of this topic, you should be able to:
- differentiate between linear, angular and general motion
- explain Newton's laws of motion and relate them to sporting examples
- classify levers and describe their effects on movement
- explain how the centre of gravity affects movement

1 Motion

Motion can be:
- **linear** — motion in a straight line (e.g. tobogganing)
- **angular** — movement around a fixed point or axis (e.g. a somersault)
- **general** — movements that are a combination of linear and angular motion (e.g. when performing a javelin throw, the body moves in a straight line on the approach, but during the throwing action the arm moves in a circular motion)

2 Force

A force can be described as a 'push' or a 'pull'. It can cause a body at rest to move or cause a moving body to stop, slow down, speed up or change direction. A force can be measured in terms of:
- **size or magnitude** — this is dependent on the size and number of muscle fibres used
- **direction** — if a force is applied through the middle of an object, it will move in the same direction as the force

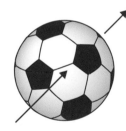
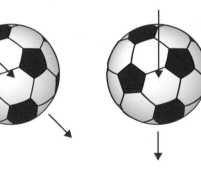

Figure 1

- **position of application** — applying a force straight through the centre of an object will result in movement in a straight line (linear motion); applying a force off-centre will result in spin (angular momentum)

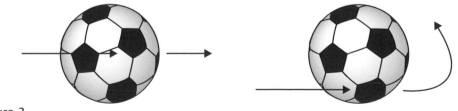

Figure 2

3 Newton's laws of motion

Make sure you can apply each of the following laws to a sporting activity.

3.1 Newton's first law of motion

A body continues in its state of rest or moves in a straight line, unless compelled to change that state or to move in a different direction by external forces exerted upon it. For example in football, the ball will remain on the penalty spot unless a force is exerted upon it.

3.2 Newton's second law of motion

The rate of momentum of a body (or the acceleration for a body of constant mass) is proportional to the force causing it and the change that takes place in the direction in which the force acts. For example, the greater the force applied to a ball, the further and faster it will go.

3.3 Newton's third law of motion

To every action there is an equal and opposite reaction. For example, when a sprinter pushes down against the blocks, the blocks push against the sprinter to an equal extent.

4 Levers

A lever depends on three main components:
- a pivot (**fulcrum**)
- the weight to be moved (**resistance**)
- a source of energy (**effort** or **force**)

In the body, the skeleton forms a system of levers that allows us to move. The joints are the fulcrums and the muscles provide the effort. A lever has two main functions:
- to increase the speed at which a body can move
- to increase the resistance against which a given effort can act

4.1 Classification of levers

Levers can be classified into three types:
- **first-order levers** — the fulcrum is between the effort and the resistance (e.g. the movement of the head and neck during flexion and extension)

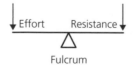

Figure 3

- **second-order levers** — the resistance lies between the fulcrum and the effort (e.g. plantar flexion of the ankle)

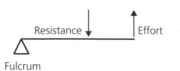

Figure 4

- **third-order levers** — responsible for the majority of movements in the human body, increasing the body's ability to move quickly rather than to move heavy weights; the effort lies between the fulcrum and the resistance (e.g. in the forearm during flexion)

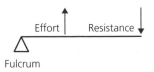

Figure 5

When the resistance arm is longer than the force arm, the lever system is at a **mechanical disadvantage**. This means that the lever system cannot move as heavy a load but can do it faster. **Mechanical advantage** is when the force arm is longer than the resistance arm. This means that the lever system can move a large load over a short distance and requires little force.

4.2 Length of lever

Most levers in the body are third-order levers, and here the resistance arm is always longer than the effort arm (mechanical disadvantage).The longer the resistance arm of the lever, the greater the speed will be at the end of it. This means that if the arm is fully extended when bowling or passing, the ball will travel with more force and therefore more speed. Extension of the arm(s) when using a cricket bat, racquet or golf club allows more force to be exerted.

5 Centre of gravity

The centre of gravity is the point of concentration of mass or, more simply, the point of balance. Because of the irregular shape of the human body, its centre of gravity is difficult to define. In addition, the body is constantly moving, so the centre of gravity will change as a result.

In general, the centre of gravity for someone adopting a standing position is in the hip region. In order to be in a balanced position, the centre of gravity needs to be in line with the base of support — your hips over your feet if you are standing. If you lower your centre of gravity, you will increase stability, while if your centre of gravity starts to move near the edge of the base of support, you will start to overbalance. Sprinters in the 'set' position have their centre of gravity right at the edge of the area of support. As they move when they hear the starting pistol, they lift their hands off the ground and become off-balanced. This allows them to fall forward, creating the speed they require to leave the blocks as quickly as possible.

Examiner's tip
The most common questions on force require knowledge of size, direction and application. Make sure that you can give specific sporting examples. For Newton's laws of motion, try to relate each law to a practical example. When identifying the type of lever, remember that the majority of levers in the body are third-order levers, except for the ankle (second) and extension of the elbow (first).

By the end of this topic, you should:
- understand the structure of a muscle and how it can contract
- know the role the motor unit plays in muscle contraction
- be able to differentiate between the three types of skeletal muscle fibre and explain their structure and relationship to physical activity

1 Skeletal muscle

Skeletal muscle is often referred to as **voluntary**, **striped** or **striated**. It is surrounded by a layer of connective tissue called the **epimysium**, which consists mainly of collagen fibres. The function of the epimysium is to provide a smooth surface against which other muscles can glide.

Skeletal muscle is made up of bundles of muscle fibres, which are enclosed in a connective tissue sheath called the **perimysium**. Each of these individual muscle fibres is made up of many smaller fibres called **myofibrils**, which are covered by a thin layer of connective tissue or **endomysium** (see Figure 6).

The epimysium, perimysium and endomysium are all connected to one another, so that when the muscle fibres contract, movement occurs through their links with the tendons and their attachment to bones at joints.

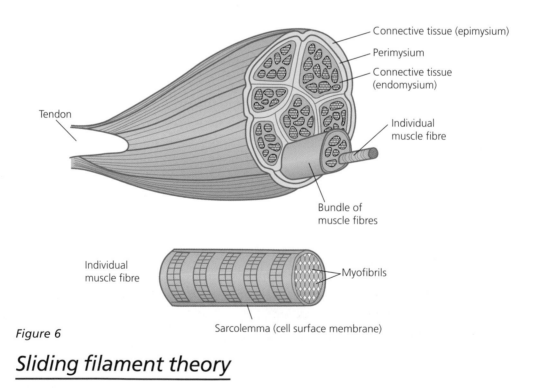

Figure 6

2 Sliding filament theory

The myofibril is the contractile unit of the muscle and runs the length of the fibre. Under a microscope, it is possible to see cross-bands or striations running across it (Figure 7).

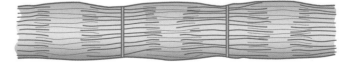

Figure 7

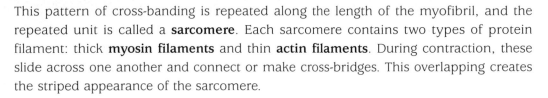

This pattern of cross-banding is repeated along the length of the myofibril, and the repeated unit is called a **sarcomere**. Each sarcomere contains two types of protein filament: thick **myosin filaments** and thin **actin filaments**. During contraction, these slide across one another and connect or make cross-bridges. This overlapping creates the striped appearance of the sarcomere.

The overlapping is made possible by the design of both the actin and the myosin. The actin has binding sites and the myosin can attach to these using tiny protein projections shaped like golf clubs. Each of these projections contains ATPase (the enzyme used to break down ATP), which provides the energy to bind the myosin cross-bridge onto the actin filament and to allow muscular contraction to take place.

The actin filament also contains two molecules called **troponin** and **tropomyosin**. These cover the binding sites of the actin and stop the myosin from forming a cross-bridge with the actin. In order to overcome this, the release of calcium from the sarcoplasmic reticulum attracts the troponin, which neutralises the tropomyosin. This frees the binding sites on the actin, allowing cross-bridges to occur.

This sliding filament theory works rather like a ratchet mechanism, where the cross-bridges attach, detach and then reattach; the net result is shortening of the sarcomere. When the sarcomere has shortened, the muscle is contracting (Figure 8).

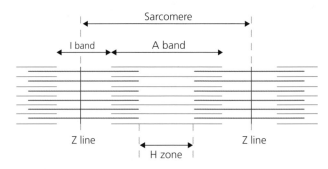

Figure 8

The Z lines move closer together. The I bands, containing only actin, get smaller, as does the H zone, which contains only myosin filaments. The A band contains both actin and myosin filaments.

3 *The motor unit*

In order for muscle to contract, it must be sent an impulse from the cerebrum or spinal cord via the nerve cells (**neurones**). This system is known as a motor unit and is illustrated in Figure 9.

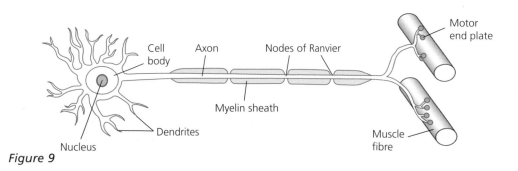

Figure 9

The **dendrites** receive impulses from other neurones and pass them on to the cell body, which in turn sorts out the information and sends an impulse down the nerve along the **axon**. These impulses are electrical, similar to currents in a wire. To protect them, an insulator called **myelin sheath**, made up of fatty material, surrounds the axon. This myelin sheath is absent at intervals along the axon, and these breaks are called the **nodes of Ranvier**. These allow the impulse to travel quickly, as it jumps from one node of Ranvier to the next. The thicker the myelin sheath, the faster the impulse is conducted.

As the impulse reaches the end of the axon, it triggers the release of **acetycholine** at the neuromuscular junction (where the axon connects with the motor end plate of the muscle).

One motor neurone stimulates between 15 and 2000 fibres within a muscle. Together, the motor neurone and the fibres it stimulates make up a motor unit.

3.1 The all-or-nothing law

The minimum amount of stimulation required to start a contraction is called the threshold. If an impulse is equal to or more than the threshold, all the muscle fibres in a motor unit will contract. However, if the impulse is less than the threshold, no muscle action will occur. As such, the motor unit exhibits an all-or-nothing response.

3.2 Gradation of contraction

The force exerted by a muscle is dependent on three factors:
- **Recruitment**. The more motor units recruited, the greater the number of muscle fibres that contract, thus increasing the force that can be produced.
- **Frequency**. The greater the frequency of stimuli, the greater the tension developed by the muscle. This is often referred to as **wave summation** — the repeated activation of a motor neurone stimulating a given muscle fibre. This means that the muscle becomes more tense. If the stimuli occur infrequently, the calcium concentration in the sarcomere returns to resting level before the arrival of the next stimulus. When the stimuli occur frequently, not all the calcium released in response to the first one is taken back into the sarcoplasmic reticulum. As a result, summation occurs (see Figure 10).

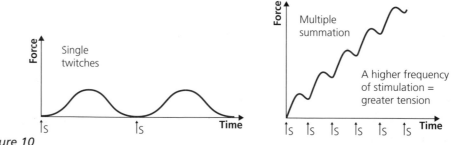

Figure 10

- **Timing**. If all the motor units are stimulated at exactly the same time, maximum force can be applied. This is sometimes referred to as **spatial summation** or **synchronisation**.

4 *Types of muscle fibre*

There are three main types of muscle fibre:
- type I (slow oxidative)
- type IIa (fast oxidative glycolytic)
- type IIb (fast glycolytic)

Our skeletal muscles contain a mixture of all three types of fibre, but not in equal proportions. This mix is mainly genetically determined. The fibres are grouped into motor units, and only one type of fibre can be found in one particular unit.

The relative proportion of each fibre type varies in the same muscles of different people. For example:

● In an elite endurance athlete, there will be a greater proportion of slow-oxidative fibres in the leg muscles.
● In the elite sprinter, there will a greater proportion of fast-glycolytic fibres in the leg muscles.

Postural muscles tend to have a greater proportion of slow-oxidative fibres, as they are involved in maintaining body position over a long period of time.

All three fibre types have specific characteristics that allow them to perform their role successfully. These are summarised in the table below.

Characteristic	Type I	Type IIa	Type IIb
Contraction speed	Slow	Fast	Fast
Motor neurone size	Small	Large	Large
Force produced	Low	High	High
Fatiguability	Low (long duration)	Medium (lower duration)	High (easily fatigued)
Mitochondria density	High	Lower	Low
Myoglobin level	High	Lower	Low
Glycogen store	Low	Medium	High
Capillaries	Dense network	Medium density	Low density
Aerobic capacity	High	Medium	Low
Anaerobic capacity	Low	Medium	High
Elasticity	Low	Medium	High

4.1 Effect of training on fibre types

Although fibre types appear to be genetically determined, it is possible to increase the size of muscle fibres through training. This increase in size (**hypertrophy**) is caused by an increase in the number and size of myofibrils per fibre, with a consequent increase in the amount of protein (**myosin**). As a result, there will be greater strength in the muscle.

Examiner's tip

The sliding filament theory is required only for the AQA specification.

Questions on the characteristics of fibre type ask for structural and/or functional characteristics. Make sure that you can distinguish between these and give examples. Also ensure you can relate the type of fibre to specific sports performers.

TOPIC 4 The heart

By the end of this topic, you should be able to:

- explain how blood moves around the body
- describe the link between the cardiac cycle and the conduction system of the heart
- define stroke volume, heart rate and cardiac output, and give resting values
- explain the relationship between stroke volume, heart rate and cardiac output and describe what happens to these during both low- and high-intensity exercise
- explain neural, hormonal and intrinsic control of heart rate
- evaluate the impact of different types of physical activity on the heart and understand coronary heart disease, heart attack and angina

1 Structure of the heart

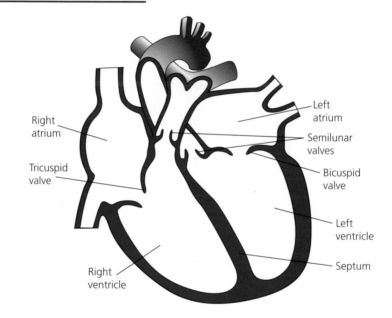

Figure 11

The heart comprises the following:

- **Aorta** — this carries oxygenated blood to the body.
- **Blood vessels** — several blood vessels are attached to the heart. They bring either oxygenated or deoxygenated blood to the heart and take it away.
- **Chambers** — the heart is divided into two parts by a muscular wall called the **septum**; each part contains an **atrium** and a **ventricle**. The atria are small and do not require much force, as they simply push blood into the ventricles. The ventricles have much thicker muscular walls, as they need to contract with greater force to push blood out of the heart. The left ventricle is larger than the right, as it pumps blood all round the body, whereas the right ventricle only pumps deoxygenated blood to the lungs.
- **Coronary artery** — this supplies the heart with oxygenated blood so that it can work effectively.
- **Pulmonary artery** — this carries deoxygenated blood to the lungs.
- **Pulmonary vein** — this carries oxygenated blood from the lungs into the left atrium.
- **Valves** — there are four main valves, which regulate blood flow by ensuring that it moves in only one direction. They open to allow blood to pass through and then close to prevent back-flow. The **tricuspid valve** is located between the right atrium and right ventricle and the **bicuspid valve** lies between the left atrium and the left

ventricle. The **semilunar valves** can be found between the right and left ventricles and the pulmonary artery and aorta respectively.

● **Vena cava** — this carries deoxygenated blood from the body to the right atrium.

2 Transportation of blood around the body

There are two types of circulation:

● **pulmonary** — deoxygenated blood is carried from the heart to the lungs, and oxygenated blood is taken back to the heart

● **systemic** — oxygenated blood is carried to the body from the heart, and deoxygenated blood returns from the body to the heart

These are illustrated in Figure 12.

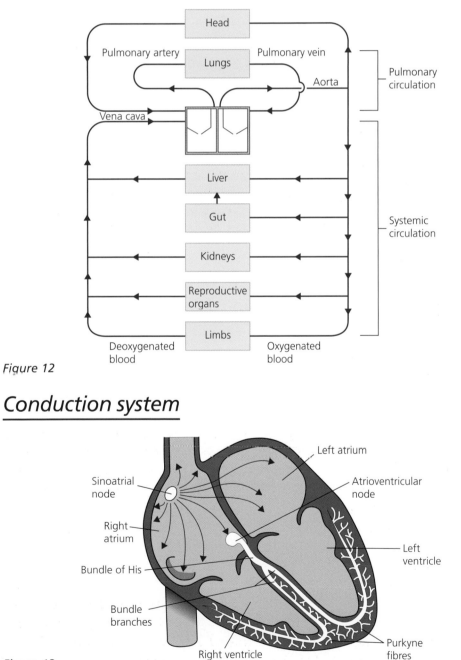

Figure 12

3 Conduction system

Figure 13

When the heart beats, the blood needs to flow through it in a controlled manner, in through the atria and out through the ventricles. Heart muscle is described as being **myogenic**, as the beat starts in the heart muscle itself with an electrical signal in the **sinoatrial node** (pacemaker). This electrical signal then spreads through the heart in what is often described as a **wave of excitation** (similar to a Mexican wave).

From the sinoatrial node, the electrical signal spreads through the walls of the atria, causing them to contract and forcing blood into the ventricles. The signal then passes through the **atrioventricular (AV) node** found in the **atrioventricular septum** and down through some specialised fibres that form the **bundle of His**. This is located in the septum separating the two ventricles. The bundle of His branches out into two bundle branches and then into smaller bundles called **Purkyne fibres**, which spread throughout the ventricles, causing them to contract.

4 Cardiac cycle

The emptying and filling of the heart (the cardiac cycle) involves a number of stages, which are summarised in the table below.

Stage	Action of atria	Result	Action of ventricles	Result
Atrial systole	Walls contract	Blood forced through the bicuspid and tricuspid valves into the ventricles	Walls relax	Ventricles fill with blood
Ventricular systole	Walls relax	Blood neither enters nor leaves the atria	Walls contract	(a) No blood leaves, but the pressure of blood in the ventricles increases (b) Pressure of blood opens the semilunar valves and blood is ejected into the pulmonary artery and aorta
Ventricular diastole	Walls relax	(a) Blood enters atria but cannot pass into the ventricles as tricuspid and bicuspid valves are closed (b) Blood enters atria and passes into ventricles as the valves open	Walls relax	(a) Blood neither enters nor leaves the ventricles (b) Blood enters from atria by passive ventricular filling (not due to atrial contraction)

5 Cardiac terms

Stroke volume: the amount of blood pumped out by the left ventricle in each contraction. On average, the resting stroke volume is approximately 70 ml. Stroke volume can be determined by the following:

- **Venous return** — this is the volume of blood returning to the heart via the veins. If venous return increases, stroke volume will increase too (i.e. if more blood enters the heart, more blood goes out).

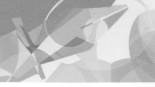

- The **elasticity of cardiac fibres** — this is concerned with the degree of stretch of cardiac tissue during the diastole phase of the cardiac cycle. The more the cardiac fibres can stretch, the greater the force of contraction will be. A greater force of contraction can increase stroke volume (this is called **Starling's Law**).
- The **contractility of cardiac tissue** (myocardium) — the greater the contractility of cardiac tissue, the greater the force of contraction. This results in an increase in stroke volume. It is also highlighted by an increase in the ejection fraction. This refers to the percentage of blood pumped out by the left ventricle per beat. An average value is 60%, but it can increase by up to 85% following a period of training:

$$\text{ejection fraction} = \frac{\text{stroke volume}}{\text{end diastolic volume}}$$

Heart rate: the number of times the heart beats per minute. On average, the resting heart rate is approximately 72 beats per minute.

Cardiac output: the amount of blood pumped out by the left ventricle per minute. It is equal to stroke volume multiplied by heart rate.

cardiac output (Q) = stroke volume (SV) × heart rate (HR)

$Q = 70 \times 72$

$Q = 5\,040$ ml (5.04 l)

5.1 Cardiac output, stroke volume, heart rate and exercise

Regular aerobic training results in hypertrophy of the cardiac muscle, i.e. the heart gets physically bigger. This has an important effect on stroke volume, heart rate and therefore cardiac output. A bigger heart enables more blood to be pumped out per beat (i.e. stroke volume). In more complex language, the **end diastolic volume** of the ventricle increases. If the ventricle can contract with more force and thus push out more blood, the heart does not have to beat as often, so the resting heart rate decreases. This is known as **bradycardia**. This increase in stroke volume and decrease in resting heart rate means that cardiac output at rest remains unchanged. However, this is not the case during exercise: an increase in heart rate coupled with an increase in stroke volume results in an increase in cardiac output.

The following table shows the differences in cardiac output (to the nearest litre) in a trained and an untrained individual, both at rest and during exercise. The individual in this example is aged 18, so the maximum heart rate will be 202 beats per minute. (Maximum heart rate is calculated as 220 minus your age.)

	SV	×	HR	=	Q
Untrained, at rest	70	×	72	=	5 litres
Untrained, during exercise	120	×	202	=	24 litres
Trained, at rest	85	×	60	=	5 litres
Trained, during exercise	170	×	202	=	34 litres

This increase in cardiac output has huge benefits for the trained person, as more blood, and therefore more oxygen, can be transported to the working muscles. In addition, when the body starts to exercise, the distribution of blood flow changes. This means that a much higher proportion of blood passes to the working muscles, and less passes to non-essential organs.

Stroke volume increases as exercise intensity increases. However, this is only the case up to 40–60% of maximum effort. Once a performer reaches this point, stroke volume plateaus (Figure 14). One explanation for this is that the increased heart rate near maximum effort results in a shorter diastolic phase. The ventricles do not have as much time to fill up with blood, so cannot pump as much out.

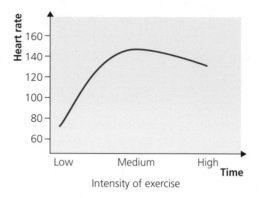

Figure 14

5.2 Control of heart rate

Heart rate is governed by three factors: **neural control**, **hormonal control** and **intrinsic control**.

5.2a Neural control

Neural control involves the autonomic nervous system. This consists of the **sympathetic system**, which stimulates the heart to beat faster, and the **parasympathetic system**, which returns the heart to its resting level. These two systems are coordinated by the **cardiac control centre**, located in the **medulla oblongata** of the brain. The cardiac control centre is stimulated by:

- **chemoreceptors** (which detect an increase in carbon dioxide)
- **baroreceptors** (which detect an increase in blood pressure)
- **proprioceptors** (which detect an increase in muscle movement)

This centre then sends an impulse through either the sympathetic or parasympathetic systems to the sinoatrial (SA) node of the heart.

5.2b Hormonal control

Adrenalin and noradrenalin stimulate the SA node (pacemaker) and increase both the speed and force of muscle contraction.

5.2c Intrinsic control

During exercise, the heart becomes warmer, so heart rate increases. Similarly, a drop in temperature reduces heart rate. In addition, venous return increases during exercise, which stretches the cardiac muscle, stimulating the SA node and, in turn, increasing heart rate and the force of contraction (Starling's Law). As a result, stroke volume increases.

It used to be thought that while exercising at a steady level, the body reached a steady state where the heart rate remained the same. However, by monitoring heart rate more closely, new research has shown that it does not stay the same but instead slowly climbs. This is known as **cardiovascular drift**.

5.3 Graphic representation of heart rate

Exam questions often ask for a graphic representation of heart rate. The intensity of the exercise will determine the type of graph required. Figure 15 shows some examples.

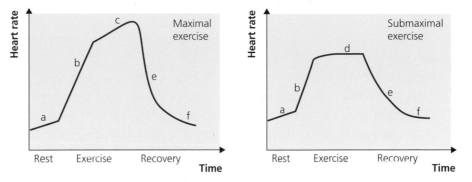

a = *anticipatory rise* due to hormonal action of adrenalin

b = *sharp rise* in heart rate due mainly to anaerobic work

c = *heart rate* continues to rise due to maximal workloads stressing the anaerobic systems

d = *steady state* as the athlete is able to meet the oxygen demand

e = *rapid decline* in heart rate as soon as the exercise stops

f = *slower recovery* as body systems return to resting levels

Figure 15

6 Impact of physical activity on the cardiovascular system

Physical activity can help to improve the health of the heart muscle, making it stronger. In turn, this will enable the heart to pump more blood around the body. There are many heart diseases that are related to a lack of exercise, which include **coronary heart disease**, **heart attack** and **angina**.

6.1 Coronary heart disease

Studies often show that regular physical activity and the avoidance of high-fat foods are the two most successful means of preventing heart disease. Medical experts recommend that individuals should be physically active for approximately 30 minutes every day. Moderate aerobic exercise can reduce cholesterol and lipid levels, including low-density lipoprotein (LDL — 'bad' cholesterol). Aerobic exercise can also increase levels of high-density lipoprotein (HDL — 'good' cholesterol), which is associated with a decrease in coronary heart disease.

Resistance training, for example lifting weights, has also been shown to lower heart rate and blood pressure after exercise. This will reduce the risk of heart disease.

6.2 Heart attack

Coronary heart disease can lead to a heart attack, when part of the heart muscle dies because it has been starved of oxygen. Regular aerobic exercise, such as brisk walking, jogging, swimming and cycling, can help prevent heart attacks.

6.3 Angina

Angina is chest pain or discomfort that occurs when the heart muscle does not receive enough oxygen because of reduced blood flow. It is usually a symptom of coronary heart disease. Exercises that train and strengthen the chest muscles will help angina.

Examiner's tip

Remember that pulmonary circulation is heart ⟶ lungs ⟶ heart, and systemic circulation is heart ⟶ body ⟶ heart. Questions often relate the conduction system to the cardiac cycle, so do not just learn them as two separate systems. Always label your graphs and explain your labels to make sure that what you have drawn is clear to the examiner. Questions on neural control of the heart are often written in relation to an increase in carbon dioxide.

5 The vascular system

By the end of this topic, you should be able to:
- explain pulmonary and systematic circulation in relation to the various blood vessels
- describe the venous return mechanisms
- understand how blood is redistributed during exercise (vascular shunt)
- describe how oxygen and carbon dioxide are transported in the blood
- describe how smoking affects the transportation of oxygen
- describe the effect a warm-up and cool-down has on the vascular system
- explain what is meant by blood pressure and velocity, and relate these terms to specific blood vessels
- explain the changes that occur in blood pressure during exercise
- evaluate the impact of physical activity on the vascular system

1 Constituents of blood

- **Plasma** is a pale yellow fluid consisting of water (90 %), proteins (8 %) and salts (2 %).
- **Red blood cells** contain an iron-rich protein called **haemoglobin** that combines with oxygen and transports it in the blood.
- **White blood cells** fight infection and disease.
- **Platelets** are responsible for clotting the blood.

2 Types and structure of blood vessels

The vascular system consists of five different blood vessels that carry the blood from the heart, distribute it round the body and then return it to the heart. The order in which the blood flows through the vascular system is as follows:

Heart ⟶ Arteries ⟶ Arterioles ⟶ Capillaries ⟶ Venules ⟶ Veins ⟶ Heart

Arteries, arterioles, venules and veins all have a similar structure:
- The **tunica externa** is the outer layer, containing collagen fibres.
- The **tunica media** is the middle layer, made up of elastic fibres and smooth muscle.
- The **tunica interna** is the inner layer, made up of thin epithelial cells, which are smooth to reduce friction.

Feature	Arteries	Capillaries	Veins
Tunica externa	Present	Absent	Present
Tunica media	Thick with many elastic fibres	Absent	Thinner than in an artery
Tunica interna	Present	Present	Present
Size of lumen	Small	Microscopic	Large
Valves	Absent	Absent	Present

3 Venous return

Venous return is the return of blood to the right side of the heart via the veins. Up to 70 % of the total blood volume is contained in the veins at rest. This means that a large amount of blood can be returned to the heart when needed.

The heart can only pump out as much blood as it receives, so cardiac output is dependent on venous return. A rapid increase in venous return enables a significant increase in stroke volume and therefore cardiac output. Veins have a large lumen and offer little resistance to blood flow. By the time blood enters the veins, blood pressure is low. Active mechanisms are needed to ensure venous return, including:

- the **skeletal muscle pump** — when muscles contract and relax, they change shape. Consequently, muscles press on nearby veins, causing a pumping effect and squeezing the blood towards the heart.
- the **respiratory pump** — when muscles contract and relax during the inspiration and expiration process, pressure changes occur in the thoracic and abdominal cavities. These pressure changes compress the nearby veins and assist the flow of blood back to the heart.
- **valves** — it is important that blood in the veins only flows in one direction. The presence of valves ensures that this happens. Once the blood has passed through the valves, they close to prevent the blood flowing back.
- **gravity** — this assists the flow of blood from body parts above the heart.
- the **smooth muscle** within the walls of the veins — it helps squeeze the blood back to the heart

4 *Vasomotor control*

Both blood pressure and blood flow are controlled by the vasomotor centre, located in the medulla oblongata of the brain. The vasomotor centre is stimulated by **chemoreceptors** (which detect increases in CO_2) and **baroreceptors** (which respond to increases in blood pressure). Blood flow is then redistributed through:

- **vasodilation**, where the blood vessels surrounding the muscles widen, thus increasing blood flow
- **vasoconstriction**, where the blood vessels surrounding non-essential organs (such as liver) narrow, thus decreasing blood flow

4.1 Vascular shunt

During exercise, vasodilation occurs in order to increase blood flow and supply the extra oxygen required by the working muscles. At the same time, vasoconstriction occurs in the arterioles, supplying non-essential organs. This redirection of blood flow is referred to as the **vascular shunt**.

Pre-capillary sphincters also aid blood redistribution. These are tiny rings of muscle located at the openings of capillaries. When they contract, the blood flow is restricted through the capillary; when they relax, blood flow is increased. During exercise, the capillary networks supplying skeletal muscle relax the pre-capillary sphincters in order to increase blood flow and thereby saturate the tissues with oxygen.

4.2 Transportation of oxygen and carbon dioxide

Oxygen plays a major role in energy production; a reduction in the amount of oxygen in the body will have a detrimental impact on performance. During exercise, when oxygen diffuses into the capillaries supplying the skeletal muscles, 3% dissolves into plasma and 97% combines with haemoglobin to form **oxyhaemoglobin**. At the tissues, oxygen dissociates from the haemoglobin due to the lower pressure of oxygen that exists there. In the muscle, oxygen is stored by myoglobin. This has a higher affinity for oxygen, and will store it in the **mitochondria** until it is used by the muscles. The mitochondria are the centres in the muscle where aerobic respiration takes place.

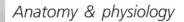

Carbon dioxide can be transported around the body in the following ways:

- 70 % can be transported in the blood as **hydrogen carbonate (bicarbonate) ions**. The carbon dioxide produced by the muscles as a waste product diffuses into the bloodstream where it combines with water to form **carbonic acid**. The weakness of the carbonic acid results in its dissociation into hydrogen carbonate (bicarbonate) ions.
- 23 % combines with haemoglobin to form **carbaminohaemoglobin**.
- 7 % dissolves in plasma.

4.2a Smoking and the transportation of oxygen

Smoking reduces the amount of oxygen available in the body. As already discussed, oxygen is transported by combining with haemoglobin. However, the high levels of carbon monoxide inhaled through smoking can affect this.

Carbon monoxide has a greater affinity for haemoglobin than oxygen (200 to 300 times greater). This means that the level of carbon monoxide absorbed in the blood from the lungs will increase while the level of oxygen decreases. Increased levels of carbon monoxide in the blood will also reduce the amount of oxygen that is released from the blood into the muscles, impacting on performance.

In addition, smoke inhalation increases resistance in the airways (often through the swelling of mucous membranes), and therefore reduces the amount of oxygen absorbed into the blood.

4.3 Warm-up and cool-down periods

Warming up helps to prepare the body for exercise. During the warm-up period, the vasomotor centre ensures that vasodilation occurs, so that more blood (and, therefore, oxygen) is transported to the working muscles (due to the increase in cardiac output). The warm-up allows for an increase in body and muscle temperature, which:

- facilitates an increase in the transportation of the enzymes necessary for energy systems and muscle contraction
- decreases blood viscosity, improving blood flow to the working muscles
- enables oxygen to dissociate from haemoglobin more quickly

The warm-up period also decreases the **onset of blood lactic acid (OBLA)**.

Cooling down (such as a gentle jog) is an activity that keeps the heart rate elevated, allowing the body to take in extra oxygen in order to reduce recovery time. An active cool-down period keeps the respiratory and skeletal muscle pumps working, preventing blood pooling in the veins and maintaining venous return. The capillaries remain dilated so that the muscles can be flushed with oxygenated blood. This increases the removal of lactic acid and carbon dioxide.

5 *Blood pressure*

Blood pressure is the force exerted by the blood against the blood vessel wall and can be referred to as **blood flow multiplied by resistance**.

Contraction of the ventricles creates a high-pressure pulse of blood — **systolic pressure**. The lower pressure as the ventricles relax is **diastolic pressure**.

Blood pressure is measured at the brachial artery (in the upper arm) using a **sphygmo-manometer**. A typical reading is:

$$\text{Systolic pressure} \diagdown \frac{120}{80} \diagup \text{Diastolic pressure} \quad \text{mmHg (millimetres of mercury)}$$

Blood pressure is different in the various blood vessels and is largely dependent on the distance of the blood vessel from the heart.

Blood pressure			
Arteries	**Arterioles**	**Capillaries**	**Veins**
High and in pulses	Not quite as high	Pressure drops throughout the capillary network	Low

6 Blood velocity

The velocity of blood flow is related to the cross-sectional area of the vessels it is passing through: the smaller the cross-sectional area, the faster the blood flows. Although the capillaries are the smallest of the blood vessels, the fact that there are so many of them means that their total cross-sectional area is much greater than that of the aorta. This means that the flow of blood is slower in the capillaries and this allows enough time for efficient exchanges with the tissues.

6.1 Effect of exercise on blood pressure and blood volume

During exercise, changes in blood pressure depend on the type and intensity of the activity being performed. Systolic pressure increases during aerobic exercise, due to both an increase in cardiac output and the vasoconstriction of arterioles that occurs during the redirection of blood flow to the working muscles. Diastolic pressure remains constant. When exercise reaches a steady state and heart rate plateaus, systolic pressure can decrease because of vasodilation in the same arterioles. This reduces total peripheral resistance and lowers mean blood pressure (the average value of systolic and diastolic pressures) to just above resting levels.

During isometric work, diastolic pressure also increases, due to an increased resistance on blood vessels caused by the contracting muscle. A decrease in blood volume occurs during exercise, when plasma moves out of the capillaries and into the surrounding tissues. After a period of training, blood volume increases, mainly due to an increase in the volume of blood plasma and a small increase in red blood cells.

7 Impact of physical activity on the vascular system

Regular endurance activity can impact on the vascular system. Arterial walls become more elastic, which means they can cope with higher fluctuations in blood pressure. There is also an increase in the number of capillaries surrounding the lungs and the muscles, and a small increase in red blood cells, all of which improve oxygen transportation.

Research shows that regular aerobic activity can help prevent vascular diseases such as **arteriosclerosis** and **atherosclerosis**:

- Arteriosclerosis is more commonly referred to as 'hardening of the arteries' and can contribute to strokes and heart attacks. The walls of the arteries thicken, harden and lose their elasticity. Lack of physical activity is a risk factor for this condition.
- Atherosclerosis is a type of arteriosclerosis. It is a common disorder, when fat and cholesterol collect along the wall of the arteries. They form a hard substance called plaque, which can cause the arteries to become narrow and less flexible and make it increasingly difficult for blood to flow.

Examiner's tip

Popular questions on the vascular system cover the redistribution of blood flow and how it is achieved (vascular shunt), as well as venous return and the mechanisms associated with it. However, with the latter, AQA does *not* award marks for gravity as a mechanism, but OCR does.

6 The respiratory system

By the end of this topic, you should be able to:

- describe the mechanics of breathing at rest and during exercise
- identify different lung volumes and capacities and interpret them on a spirometer trace, giving values at rest and during exercise
- describe the process of gaseous exchange between the alveoli and the blood, and between the blood and the muscle cells
- explain the principles of diffusion and the importance of partial pressures
- explain the difference in oxygen (A-VO$_2$ diff) and carbon dioxide content between alveolar air and pulmonary blood
- explain the increased diffusion gradient and the accelerated dissociation of oxyhaemoglobin
- explain the effects of altitude training on the respiratory system
- explain how breathing is controlled
- describe how physical activity can have an impact on the respiratory system (to include an understanding of smoking and asthma)

1 Structure of the lungs

As Figure 16 shows, the lungs are protected by the ribcage and found in the thorax. The right lung is slightly larger and has three sections, called **lobes**; the left lung has two lobes. Each lung is surrounded by a **pleura** — a double layer of membrane that contains lubricating pleural fluid to reduce friction. The lungs are separated from the abdomen by the **diaphragm**, which is a large sheet of skeletal muscle.

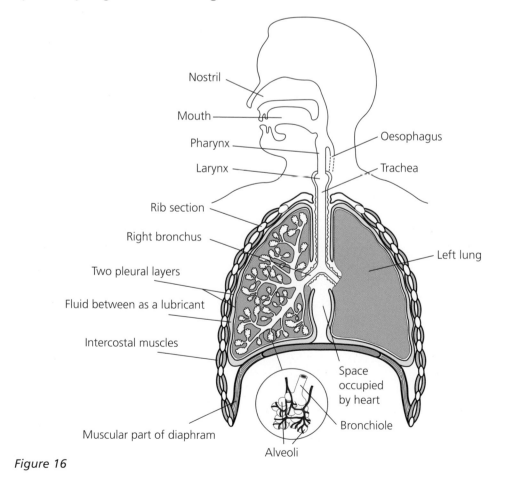

Nostril

Mouth

Pharynx

Larynx

Oesophagus

Trachea

Rib section

Right bronchus

Two pleural layers

Fluid between as a lubricant

Intercostal muscles

Left lung

Space occupied by heart

Bronchiole

Muscular part of diaphram

Alveoli

Figure 16

Air, containing oxygen, travels from the atmosphere, passing through several structures before it reaches the bloodstream. The order in which it travels is as follows:

nose ⟶ pharynx ⟶ trachea ⟶ bronchus (right or left) ⟶ bronchioles ⟶ alveoli

The **alveoli** are responsible for the exchange of gases between the lungs and the blood. Their structure is designed to help this process:

- Their walls are very thin (only one cell thick) and are supplied by a dense capillary network.
- They have a huge surface area, which allows for a greater uptake of oxygen.

2 Mechanics of breathing

Air always moves from an area of high pressure to an area of low pressure. The greater the difference in pressure, the faster the air will flow. Changing the volume of the thoracic cavity can alter the pressure of air in the lungs:

- Reducing the volume increases the pressure within the alveoli, forcing air out.
- Increasing the volume decreases the pressure within the alveoli, drawing air in.

Inspiration increases the volume of the thoracic cavity through the contraction of muscles. Expiration reduces the volume of the thoracic cavity.

2.1 Respiratory muscles

Ventilation phase	Muscles used during breathing at rest	Muscles used during exercise
Inspiration	Diaphragm External intercostals	Diaphragm External intercostals Sternocleidomastoid Scalenes Pectoralis major
Expiration	Passive — diaphragm and external intercostals just relax	Internal intercostals Abdominals

2.2 Respiratory volumes

Lung volume or capacity	Definition	Average values at rest	Average values during exercise	Changes during exercise
Tidal volume	Volume of air breathed in or out per breath	0.5 l	2.8 l	Increase
Inspiratory reserve volume	Volume of air that can be forcibly inspired after a normal breath	3.1 l	1.0 l	Decrease
Expiratory reserve volume	Volume of air that can be forcibly expired after a normal breath	1.2 l	1.0 l	Slight decrease
Residual volume	Volume of air that remains in the lungs after maximum expiration	1.2 l	1.2 l	Remains the same

Lung volume or capacity	Definition	Average values at rest	Average values during exercise	Changes during exercise
Vital capacity	Volume of air forcibly expired after maximum inspiration in one breath	4.8l	4.8l	Remains the same
Minute ventilation	Volume of air breathed in or out per minute	6.0l	110.0l	Increases
Total lung capacity	Vital capacity + residual volume	6.0l	6.0l	Remains the same

These lung volumes can be interpreted on a spirometer trace like the one below.

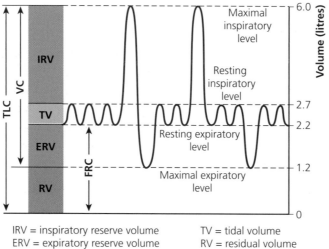

IRV = inspiratory reserve volume   TV = tidal volume
ERV = expiratory reserve volume   RV = residual volume
TLC = total lung capacity   VC = vital capacity
FRC = functional residual capacity

Figure 17

3 Gaseous exchange

3.1 Gaseous exchange at the lungs

Gaseous exchange refers to the replenishment of oxygen in the blood and the removal of carbon dioxide. The term '**partial pressure**' is often used when describing the gaseous exchange process.

In simple terms, all gases exert a pressure. Oxygen makes up only a small part of air (approximately 21 %), so it therefore exerts a partial pressure. As gases flow from an area of high pressure to an area of low pressure, it is important that, as air moves from the alveoli to the blood and then to the muscle, the partial pressure of oxygen in each needs to be successively lower.

The partial pressure of oxygen in the alveoli (105 mmHg) is higher than that in the capillary blood vessels (40 mmHg). This is because oxygen has been removed by the working muscles, so its concentration in the blood is lower and therefore so is its partial pressure. The difference between any two pressures is referred to as the **concentration/diffusion gradient**, and the steeper this gradient, the faster diffusion will be. Oxygen diffuses from the alveoli into the blood until the pressure is equal in both.

The movement of carbon dioxide occurs in the reverse order. The partial pressure of carbon dioxide in the blood entering the alveolar capillaries is higher (45 mmHg) than in the alveoli (40 mmHg), so carbon dioxide diffuses from the blood into the alveoli until the pressure is equal in both.

3.2 Gaseous exchange at the tissues (internal respiration)

In order for diffusion to occur, the partial pressure of oxygen has to be lower at the tissues than in the blood. In the capillary membranes surrounding the muscle, the partial pressure of oxygen is 40 mmHg, and it is 105 mmHg in the blood. This lower partial pressure allows oxygen to diffuse from the blood into the muscle until equilibrium is reached. Conversely, the partial pressure of carbon dioxide in the blood (40 mmHg) is lower than in the tissues (45 mmHg), so again diffusion occurs and carbon dioxide moves into the blood to be transported to the lungs.

3.3 Arteriovenous difference

This is the difference between the oxygen content of the arterial blood arriving at the muscles and that of the venous blood leaving the muscles. At rest, the arteriovenous difference is low, as not much oxygen is required by the muscles. However, during exercise the muscles need much more oxygen from the blood, so the arteriovenous difference is high. This increase will affect gaseous exchange at the alveoli, due to the high concentration of carbon dioxide returning to the heart in the venous blood and the presence of less oxygen. This will increase the diffusion gradient for both gases.

Training also increases the arteriovenous difference, as trained performers are able to extract a greater amount of oxygen from the blood.

3.4 The oxyhaemoglobin dissociation curve

The relationship of oxygen and haemoglobin is often represented by the oxyhaemoglobin dissociation curve, shown in Figure 18.

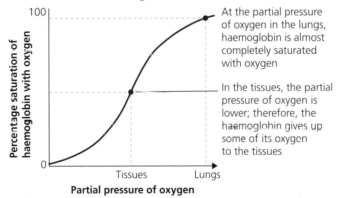

Figure 18

From this curve, you can see that in the lungs there is almost full saturation of haemoglobin, but at the tissues the partial pressure of oxygen is lower. This means that there is less oxygen in the tissues, so haemoglobin has to give up some of its oxygen and therefore is no longer fully saturated.

During exercise, this s-shaped curve shifts to the right; when muscles require more oxygen, the dissociation of oxygen from haemoglobin in the blood capillaries to the muscle tissue occurs more readily.

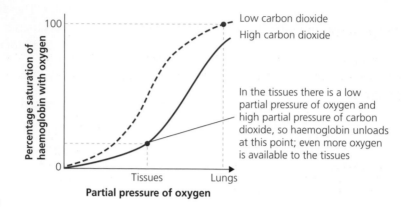

Figure 19

Four factors are responsible for this increase in the dissociation of oxygen from haemoglobin:

- a decrease in the partial pressure of oxygen in the muscle
- an increase in temperature in the blood and muscle
- an increase in carbon dioxide during exercise, which increases the carbon dioxide diffusion gradient
- an increase in acidity (caused by exercise) — more lactic acid lowers the pH in the body (Bohr effect)

4 Changes to the respiratory system

4.1 Altitude and the respiratory system

At both sea level and altitude, the percentage of oxygen within air is the same. However, the partial pressure of oxygen drops as altitude increases, usually by up to 50 % at an altitude of 5 000 m. This causes a reduction in the diffusion gradient between the air and the lungs, and between the alveoli and the blood. Therefore haemoglobin is not fully saturated, and the blood has less capacity for carrying oxygen. As less oxygen is delivered to working muscles, there is an earlier onset of fatigue, resulting in a decrease in performance of aerobic activities.

The body adapts to a relative lack of oxygen by increasing the concentration of red blood cells and haemoglobin. It is claimed that when athletes who have trained at high altitude participate in competitions at lower altitudes, they still have a higher concentration of red blood cells for 10–14 days, giving them a competitive advantage. A higher concentration of red blood cells allows more oxygen to be supplied to the muscles, resulting in higher performance.

Disadvantages of altitude training include:

- financial expense
- altitude sickness
- difficult to train due to the lack of oxygen
- detraining — training intensity has to reduce when the performer first trains at altitude because of the decreased availability of oxygen
- benefits can be quickly lost on return to sea level

4.2 Control of ventilation

Breathing is controlled by the nervous system, which automatically increases or decreases the rate, depth and rhythm of breathing. The whole process is summarised in Figure 20.

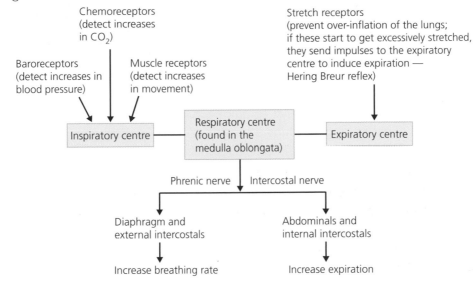

Figure 20

5 Impact of physical activity on the respiratory system

During endurance training, the body makes adaptations that contribute to an improvement in lung function:

- Small increases in lung volume occur due to an increase in the efficiency of the respiratory muscles, namely the diaphragm and external intercostals.
- The exchange of gases at the alveoli becomes more efficient, due to an increase in surface area of the alveoli and increased density of the capillaries surrounding the alveoli.
- There is an improvement in the transport of respiratory gases. Blood volume increases, mainly due to a rise in blood plasma volume, but there is also a slight increase in red blood cells, which leads to an increase in haemoglobin.
- There is an improvement in the uptake of oxygen by the muscles due to an increase in myoglobin content and mitochondrial density within the muscle cell.

5.1 Asthma

Asthma is a chronic disease where the walls of the airway occasionally constrict (get smaller) and become inflamed. This makes them sensitive and they can react to allergies or environmental stimulants such as cold/warm air, stress or exercise. When there is a reaction, the airways become narrower and less air gets to the lungs. This can cause wheezing, shortness of breath, chest tightness and coughing.

Regular physical activity can help in managing the symptoms of asthma:
- Aerobic exercise can increase lung capacity.
- In swimming, the warm humid environment is unlikely to trigger an attack.

Scuba diving is the only sport not recommended for asthma sufferers.

5.2 Smoking

Smoking has many effects on the body's respiratory system:

- High levels of carbon monoxide from smoking reduce the amount of oxygen absorbed into the blood from the lungs. Carbon monoxide in the blood also reduces the amount of oxygen that is released from the blood into the muscles.
- Smoke inhalation increases airways resistance, therefore reducing the amount of oxygen absorbed into the blood.
- Smoking causes chronic (or long-term) swelling of mucous membranes, which also leads to increased airways resistance.

Research suggests that regular aerobic exercise may have a beneficial effect in helping an individual to stop smoking, inducing biochemical changes in the body that can increase mental alertness and decrease stress levels. Such exercise can also increase the brain's endorphin levels, which can help produce a state of relaxation and wellbeing.

Examiner's tip

Questions about control of ventilation often refer to how an increase in carbon dioxide can affect breathing. Always describe the work of receptors in detail. Saying that chemoreceptors detect a change in chemicals during exercise is not accurate enough for a mark. Instead, say that chemoreceptors detect an increase in *carbon dioxide* during exercise.

TOPIC 7 Nutrition

By the end of this topic, you should be able to:
- identify the seven classes of food, and highlight types of food that fall into these categories
- identify the exercise-related function for each type of food
- describe a balanced diet and the energy balance of food, and relate this to your own practical activity
- identify the difference in diet composition between endurance athletes and power athletes
- identify the percentage body fat/body composition and body mass index (BMI) as measures of nutritional suitability
- understand the limitations in trying to define obesity

1 A balanced diet

No single food can cover all our nutritional needs, so a balanced diet involves eating a wide variety of foods. There are seven main classes of food, each with their own nutritional characteristics:
- carbohydrates
- fats
- proteins
- vitamins
- minerals
- fibre
- water

A balanced diet should contain 15% protein, 30% fat and 55% carbohydrate. During exercise, this percentage needs to change in favour of carbohydrates. Sports nutritionists recommend 10–15% protein, 20–25% fat and 60–75% carbohydrate.

1.1 Carbohydrates

There are two types of carbohydrate:
- **Simple carbohydrates** are easily digested by the body. They are found in fruits, processed foods and anything containing refined sugar.
- **Complex carbohydrates** usually take longer for the body to digest. They are commonly found in nearly all plant-based foods, bread, pasta, rice and vegetables.

Carbohydrates do not just provide fuel for muscles. It is important to consider the 'glycaemic index' and release rate of different carbohydrates, and the consequence this has on when they should be consumed in relation to training. Foods with a lower glycaemic index, such as fruit, cause a slower, sustained release of glucose to the blood, whereas foods with a high glycaemic index, such as bread and potatoes, cause a rapid, temporary rise in blood glucose:
- Suitable foods to eat 3–4 hours before exercise include beans on toast, pasta or rice with a vegetable-based sauce, breakfast cereal with milk or crumpets with jam or honey.
- Suitable snacks to eat 1–2 hours before exercise include fruit smoothies, cereal bars, fruit-flavoured yoghurt and fruit.
- One hour before exercise, liquid consumption is important, through sports drinks and cordials.

1.2 Fats

Fats are made from **glycerol** and **fatty acids**, which contain the elements carbon, hydrogen and oxygen. The high carbon content of fats accounts for why they give us so much energy. Fats are stored as triglycerides and converted to free fatty acids when required. They are the main energy source used during low-intensity exercise.

Foods high in fats include butter and cheese.

1.3 Proteins

Proteins are a combination of chemicals called **amino acids**. They promote tissue growth and repair, and make enzymes, hormones and haemoglobin. Proteins tend to provide energy when glycogen and fat stores are low. However, during strenuous activities or sustained periods of exercise, proteins in the muscles may start to be broken down to provide energy.

High-protein foods include meat, fish, eggs and cheese.

1.4 Vitamins

Vitamins are needed for muscle and nerve function, tissue growth and the release of energy from foods. Excessive consumption has no beneficial effect, as vitamins cannot be stored in the body; additional amounts will be excreted in urine.

1.5 Minerals

Minerals assist in various bodily functions, for example calcium is essential for the maintenance of strong bones and teeth, and iron assists in haemoglobin formation, which enhances the transport of oxygen and therefore improves stamina.

Minerals tend to be dissolved by the body as ions and are called **electrolytes**. They facilitate the transmission of nerve impulses and enable effective muscle contraction, both of which are important during exercise.

As with vitamins, excessive consumption is unlikely to enhance performance. However, it is important not to overdose on some minerals; too much sodium (contained in salt) can result in high blood pressure.

1.6 Fibre

Fibre is important for exercise, as it can slow down the time it takes the body to break down food, resulting in a slower, more sustained release of energy.

Good sources of fibre are wholemeal bread and pasta, potatoes, nuts, seeds, fruit, vegetables and pulses.

1.7 Water

Water constitutes up to 60% of a person's body weight. It is essential for good health, carrying nutrients to cells in the body and removing waste products. It also helps to control body temperature.

When athletes start to exercise, their production of water increases and they begin to sweat (water is a by-product of the aerobic system). When sweat evaporates from the surface of the skin, it removes excess heat. The volume of water we lose depends on the external temperature, the intensity and duration of the exercise and the volume of water consumed before, during and after exercise.

Water is important to maintain optimal performance, so it is important to take on fluids regularly. Sports drinks are useful to boost glucose levels before competition, while water is needed to rehydrate during competition.

2 Energy balance of food

When we take part in physical activity, our bodies require energy, and this is obtained from our body stores or the food we eat. The amount of energy we need is dependent on the duration and type of activity.

Energy is measured in **calories**. A calorie (cal) is the amount of heat energy required to raise the temperature of 1 g of water by 1 °C. A kilocalorie (kcal) is the amount of heat required to raise the temperature of 1 kg of water by 1 °C.

The energy requirements of an individual weighing 60 kg are:

1.3 kcal per hour × 24 (hours in a day) × 60 = 1872 kcal per day

This energy requirement increases during exercise by up to 8.5 kcal per hour for each kilogram of body weight. Therefore, in a 1-hour training session the performer would require an extra 8.5 × 1 × 60 = 510 kcal.

From these calculations, it is possible to work out the energy requirements of this performer by adding the basic energy requirements (1872 kcal) to the extra energy needed for that 1-hour training session (510 kcal): 1872 + 510 = 2382 kcal.

3 Diet and performance

3.1 Eating before a competition

Food should be consumed around 3–4 hours before competing, as it needs to be digested and absorbed in order to be useful. The meal needs to be high in carbohydrates, low in fat and moderate in fibre in order to aid digestion. High levels of carbohydrate will keep blood glucose levels high throughout the duration of the competition or performance.

3.2 Diet composition of an endurance athlete versus a power athlete

In order to replenish and maintain glycogen stores, endurance athletes require a diet rich in carbohydrates. Most research suggests that they need to consume at least 6 to 10 grams of carbohydrate per kilogram of their body weight. Another key nutrient is water, in order to avoid dehydration.

Some endurance athletes manipulate their diet to maximise aerobic energy production. One method is **glycogen loading** (see page 42).

In general, endurance athletes require more carbohydrates than power athletes because they exercise for longer periods of time and need more energy. Proteins are important for power athletes, promoting tissue growth and repair. Insufficient protein intake leads to muscle breakdown.

4 *Body fat composition*

This is the physiological make-up of an individual in terms of the distribution of lean body mass and body fat. On average, men have less body fat than women (approximately 15% as opposed to 25%).

In sport, it is generally agreed that the less body fat, the better the performance. However, there are some sports with specific requirements for larger amounts of body fat, such as the defensive linesman in American football or, if we take it to the extreme, a sumo wrestler.

5 *Body mass index (BMI)*

Body mass index (BMI) is a statistical measure of the weight of a person scaled according to height and takes into account body composition. To calculate your BMI, divide your weight in kilograms by your height in metres squared. Let us take as an example a 17-year-old, who weighs 75 kg and is 1.80 m tall:

$$BMI = \frac{weight\ (kg)}{height\ (m) \times height\ (m)}$$

$$BMI = \frac{75}{1.80 \times 1.80}$$

$$BMI = 23.15$$

BMI values vary according to which book you read, but the table below is representative of most literature.

BMI	Classification
<19	Underweight
19–25	Normal
26–30	Overweight
31–40	Obese
>40	Morbidly obese

6 *Obesity*

Obesity occurs when there is an excess proportion of total body fat, usually due to energy intake being greater than energy output. An individual is considered obese if his or her body weight is 20% or more above normal weight, or when a male accumulates 25% total body fat or a female 35% total body fat.

Obesity carries an increased risk of heart disease, hypertension, high blood cholesterol, strokes and type-2 diabetes. It can also increase stress on joints and limit flexibility.

BMI is a common measure of obesity. An individual is considered obese when his or her BMI is over 30.

Examiner's tip

This is a new topic for A-level PE. Questions may ask you to compare the dietary requirement of different types of athletes, so make sure you can apply your knowledge.

TOPIC 8 — Energy systems

By the end of this topic, you should be able to:

- define energy, work and power
- explain the role of adenosine triphosphate (ATP)
- identify the main energy sources
- explain the three energy systems
- identify which energy system is used in relation to the type of exercise being performed
- describe the interchanging between thresholds during an activity
- understand onset of blood lactate accumulation (OBLA)

1 Definitions

- **energy:** the ability to perform work (joules); includes **chemical energy** (food), **kinetic energy** (movement) and **potential energy** (stored)
- **work:** force $\times$ distance (joules)
- **power:** work performed over a unit of time (watts)
- **exothermic reaction:** a reaction that releases energy
- **endothermic reaction:** a reaction that needs energy to work

2 Role of adenosine triphosphate

Adenosine triphosphate (ATP) is the only usable form of energy in the body. The energy we derive from food, such as carbohydrates, has to be converted into ATP before it can be used. ATP consists of one molecule of adenosine and three phosphates.

Enzymes are used to break down the bonds that hold ATP together, and this causes energy to be released; ATP-ase breaks down ATP into ADP + P.

The rebuilding or re-synthesising of ATP from ADP + P is an endothermic reaction. As there is only a limited store of ATP within muscle fibres, it is used up quickly (in about 3 seconds) and therefore needs to be replenished immediately. There are three energy systems that re-synthesise/replenish ATP: **ATP/PC**, the **lactic acid system** and the **aerobic system**. These are summarised below.

Energy system	ATP/PC	Lactic acid	Aerobic
Type of reaction	Anaerobic coupled	Anaerobic coupled	Aerobic
Chemical/fuel used	Phosphocreatine	Glucose	Glucose and fats
Site of reaction	Sarcoplasm	Sarcoplasm	(a) Krebs — matrix of the mitochondria (b) Electron transport chain — cristae of the mitochondria
Controlling enzyme	Creatine kinase	PFK	PFK
Energy yield	1 ATP	2 ATP	(a) 2 ATP (b) 34 ATP
By-products	None	Lactic acid	(a) Krebs — carbon dioxide (b) Electron transport chain — water
Duration	3–8 seconds	Up to 3 minutes, peaks at 1 minute	Continuous
Intensity	High, e.g. a slam-dunk in basketball	High, e.g. a 400m sprint	Submaximal, e.g. a marathon

Specific stages in the aerobic system are illustrated in Figure 21.

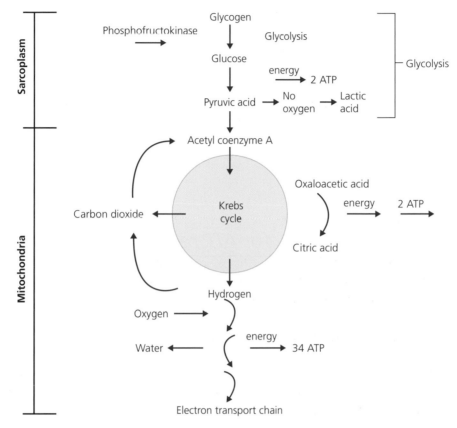

Figure 21

Energy system	Advantages	Disadvantages
ATP/PC	<ul><li>ATP can be re-synthesised rapidly using the ATP/PC system</li><li>Phosphocreatine stores can be re-synthesised quickly (30 seconds = 50% replenishment; 3 minutes = 100%)</li><li>There are no fatiguing by-products</li><li>It is possible to extend the time for the ATP/PC system through creatine supplementation</li><li>ATP can be re-synthesised quickly due to few chemical reactions</li></ul>	<ul><li>There is only a limited supply of phosphocreatine in the muscle cell; it can only last for 10 seconds</li><li>Only one mole of ATP can be re-synthesised through one mole of PC</li><li>PC re-synthesis can only take place in the presence of oxygen, i.e. the intensity of the exercise is reduced</li></ul>
Lactic acid	<ul><li>In the presence of oxygen, lactic acid can be converted back into liver glycogen or used as a fuel through oxidation into carbon dioxide and water</li><li>The system can be used for a sprint finish, i.e. to produce an extra burst of energy</li><li>More ATP can be produced — 36 ATP</li><li>There are no fatiguing by-products</li></ul>	<ul><li>Lactic acid is produced as a by-product; the accumulation of acid in the body denatures enzymes and prevents them increasing the rate at which chemical reactions take place</li></ul>

Energy system	Advantages	Disadvantages
Aerobic	• There are plenty of glycogen and triglyceride stores, so exercise can last for a long time	• This is a complicated system and therefore cannot be used straight away • It takes a while for enough oxygen to become available to meet the demands of the activity and ensure glycogen and fatty acids are broken down completely • Fatty acid transportation to the muscles is low and also requires 15% more oxygen to be broken down than glycogen.

3 Sources of energy for ATP re-synthesis

Our bodies require energy when we exercise. The more exercise we do, the more energy is required. **Phosphocreatine** is used to re-synthesise ATP in the first 10 seconds of intense exercise. It is easy to break down and stored within the muscle cell; however, its stores are limited.

Food is also used for ATP re-synthesis. The main energy foods are:

- **carbohydrates**, stored as glycogen in the muscles and the liver, and converted into glucose during exercise. During high-intensity anaerobic exercise, glycogen can be broken down without the presence of oxygen; however, it is broken down much more effectively during aerobic work when oxygen is present.
- **fats**, stored as triglycerides and converted to free fatty acids when required. At rest, two thirds of our energy requirements are met through the breakdown of fatty acids. This is because fat can produce more energy per gram than glycogen.
- **protein**. Approximately 5–10 % of energy used during exercise comes from proteins in the form of amino acids. It tends to be used when stores of glycogen are low.

Carbohydrates and fats are the main energy providers, and the intensity and duration of exercise determines which of these is used. The breakdown of fats into free fatty acids requires more oxygen than that required to break down glycogen; therefore, during high-intensity exercise, when oxygen is in limited supply, glycogen is the preferred source of energy. Fats are the favoured fuel at rest and during long, endurance-based activities.

Stores of glycogen are much smaller than stores of fat. It is important during prolonged periods of exercise not to deplete glycogen stores, as some needs to be conserved for later when the intensity could increase, for example during the last kilometre of a marathon.

4 The energy continuum

When we start any exercise, the demand for energy rises rapidly. Although all three energy systems are always working at the same time, one of them will be predominant. The intensity and duration of the activity decide which is the main energy system in use. For example:

- Jogging is a long-duration, submaximal exercise, so the aerobic system is predominant.
- A highly explosive, short-duration activity, such as the 100 metres, uses the ATP-PC system.

However, in a game there will be a mix of all three systems and the performer will move from one to another. This continual movement between the thresholds of each energy system is known as the **energy continuum**. The ATP-PC–lactic acid threshold is the point at which the ATP-PC energy system is exhausted and the lactic acid system takes over. The lactic acid–aerobic threshold is the point at which the lactic acid system is exhausted and the aerobic system takes over (see Figure 22).

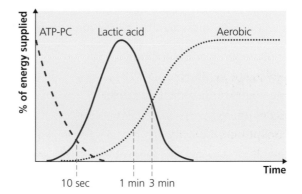

Figure 22

5 | *Onset of blood lactate accumulation (OBLA)*

The multi-stage fitness test is a good practical example to illustrate OBLA. Due to the increasing intensity of this test, the performer eventually reaches a point where energy cannot be provided aerobically. This means using anaerobic systems to re-synthesise ATP. Blood lactate levels start to increase until eventually muscle fatigue occurs and the performer slows down.

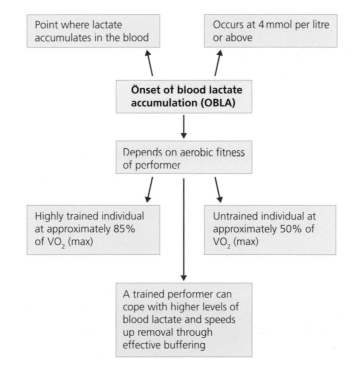

Figure 23

6 *Increasing energy stores*

By following an appropriate diet and training programme, it is possible to enhance the production of energy from each of the energy systems.

6.1 Glycogen loading

This is a form of dietary manipulation, involving the maximisation of glycogen stores. Six days before an important competition, a performer eats a diet high in protein and fats for 3 days and exercises at relatively high intensity to burn off any existing carbohydrate stores. This is followed by 3 days of a diet high in carbohydrates and some light training. This will greatly increase the stores of glycogen in the muscle.

Advantages of glycogen loading include:
- increased glycogen synthesis
- increased glycogen stores in the muscle
- delayed fatigue
- increased endurance capacity

Disadvantages of glycogen loading include:
- water retention (which results in bloating)
- weight increase
- fatigue
- irritability during the depletion phase

6.2 Creatine monohydrate

Creatine monohydrate is a supplement used to increase the amount of phosphocreatine stored in the muscles. It allows the ATP-PC system to last longer and can help improve recovery times. However, possible side effects are dehydration and slight liver damage, and studies suggest that a daily intake of 5 g or over usually ends up in urine rather than in the muscle.

6.3 Soda loading

Drinking a solution of sodium bicarbonate increases the pH of the blood and makes it more alkaline. This then increases the buffering capacity of the blood so that it can neutralise the negative effects of lactic acid.

6.4 Training

Training can improve the efficiency of each of the three energy systems, causing adaptations that will impact on ATP re-synthesis:
- ATP-PC system — sprint interval training, plyometrics and weights (90% of maximum load) will increase the stores of ATP and PC and increase enzyme activity (ATP-ase and creatine kinase).
- Lactic acid system — interval, fartlek and weight training (80% of maximum load) will cause an increase in muscle glycogen stores and increase the number of glycolytic enzymes (PFK).
- Aerobic system — continuous training will increase the stores of muscle glycogen and triglycerides and the number of oxidative enzymes.

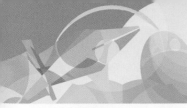

Examiner's tip

The headings listed in the left-hand column of the table on page 38 categorise the knowledge of energy systems you need. Learn the table and then make sure you have a basic overview of each system. You need to be aware of the specific stages within the aerobic system, i.e. glycolysis, the Krebs cycle and the electron transport chain. AQA papers often ask questions about energy sources, so learn them carefully.

9 The recovery process

By the end of this topic, you should be able to:

- explain how the body returns to its pre-exercise state — excess post-exercise oxygen consumption (EPOC)
- understand oxygen debt (lactacid and alactacid components) and explain the replenishment of myoglobin
- describe recovery methods

1 EPOC

During recovery, the body takes in elevated amounts of oxygen and transports it to the working muscles to maintain high rates of aerobic respiration. This surplus energy is then used to help return the body to its pre-exercise state. This is known as **excess post-exercise oxygen consumption** (EPOC). The EPOC process is summarised in Figure 24.

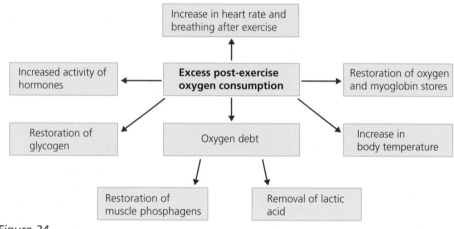

Figure 24

1.1 Oxygen debt

This is the amount of oxygen consumed during recovery, above that which would have been consumed at rest during the same time. It has two components: the **alactacid component** and the **lactacid component**.

1.1a The alactacid component (fast replenishment stage)

This is often referred to as fast replenishment and involves the restoration of ATP and phosphocreatine stores. Elevated rates of breathing continue to supply oxygen to provide the energy for ATP production and phosphocreatine replenishment. Complete restoration of phosphocreatine takes up to 3 minutes (50% of stores can be replenished after only 30 seconds), during which time approximately 3 litres of oxygen are consumed.

1.1b The lactacid component (slow replenishment stage)

This is concerned with the removal of lactic acid. It is the slower of the two processes, and full recovery may take up to an hour, depending on the intensity and duration of the exercise. Lactic acid can be removed in four ways, as outlined in the table below.

Destination of lactic acid	Approximate % lactic acid involved
Oxidation into carbon dioxide and water	65
Conversion into glycogen, then stored in muscles/liver	20
Conversion into protein	10
Conversion into glucose	5

The lactacid oxygen recovery begins as soon as lactic acid appears in the muscle cell, and will continue using breathed oxygen until recovery is complete. This can take up to 5–6 litres of oxygen in the first half hour of recovery, removing up to 50 % of the lactic acid. Figure 25 illustrates oxygen debt.

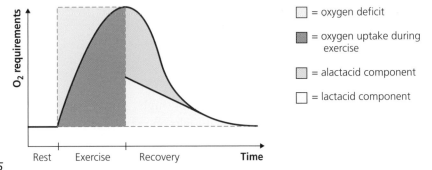

Figure 25

1.2 Myoglobin and replenishment of oxygen stores

Myoglobin has a high affinity for oxygen. It stores oxygen in the muscle and transports it from the capillaries to the mitochondria for energy provision. After exercise, oxygen stores in the mitochondria are limited. The surplus of oxygen supplied through EPOC helps replenish these stores, taking up to 2 minutes and using approximately 0.5 litres of oxygen.

1.3 Glycogen

Glycogen, as the main fuel for the aerobic system and lactic acid system, is depleted during exercise. In addition, the stores of glycogen in relation to the stores of fat are relatively small, so it is important to conserve these in order not to cross the lactate threshold. The replacement of glycogen stores occurs when an individual eats a carbohydrate meal. It has been suggested that eating a high carbohydrate meal within 1 hour of exercise will speed up the recovery process.

1.4 Increase in breathing and heart rate

This is important to assist in recovery where oxygen is required to return the body back to its pre-exercise state. However, an increase in both breathing and heart rate requires extra oxygen to provide energy for the muscles of the heart and respiratory systems.

1.5 Increased activity of hormones

The continuation of a submaximal activity, such as jogging, will keep hormonal levels elevated, and this will keep respiratory and metabolic levels high.

1.6 Increase in body temperature

When temperature remains high, breathing rates will also remain high; this will help the performer take in more oxygen during recovery. However, extra oxygen is needed to fuel this increase in temperature until the body returns to normal.

2 Methods of speeding up the recovery process

2.1 Hyperbaric chambers

A hyperbaric chamber is pressurised rather like an aeroplane (in some chambers a mask is worn). The pressure increases the amount of oxygen that can be breathed in; this means more oxygen can be diffused to the injured area. The dissolved oxygen can reduce swelling and stimulate the body's cells to repair.

2.2 Oxygen tents

Oxygen tents simulate the effects of high altitude by providing a low-oxygen environment. Performers who use them tend to train or sleep in them. They are popular with endurance athletes, as it is believed that they improve cardiovascular capacity by increasing the production of red blood cells. This in turn improves the capacity of the blood for carrying oxygen. Oxygen tents do not make a difference to the speed of the healing process, but when the performer has recovered from injury, they will have retained a level of fitness that allows them to return to their sport almost immediately.

2.3 Ice baths

Ice baths are a popular method of recovery. After a gruelling training session or match, performers immerse their body in icy water for 5 to 10 minutes. This causes the blood vessels to tighten and drains the blood out of the legs. On leaving the bath, the legs fill up with new blood that invigorates the muscles with oxygen to help the cells function better. The blood that leaves the legs takes away with it the lactic acid that has built up during the activity.

Examiner's tip

Care needs to be taken when answering questions on the recovery process. Remember that oxygen debt is not separate from EPOC, but a part of it. Questions on EPOC usually involve an explanation of key areas, namely oxygen debt (lactacid and alactacid components) and the replenishment of myoglobin. Make sure you learn these comprehensively.

By the end of this topic, you should be able to:
- build upon the principles of training covered at GCSE and apply them to the planning of a training programme
- explain the physiological effects of a warm-up and a cool-down
- describe the different types of training and relate fitness components to specific training methods

1 | *Principles of training*

In order to improve fitness, it is important to follow an effective training programme. This may include some of the following principles:
- overload (FITT)
- progression
- specificity
- reversibility
- moderation
- variance
- warm-up
- cool-down

1.1 Overload (FITT)

Overload is achieved by increasing one or more of the following:
- **frequency** — the number of times you train per week
- **intensity** — how hard you work
- **time** — the duration of the session
- **type** — the type of training

If you wish to increase aerobic fitness, it is important to increase the intensity of the exercise by training above the aerobic threshold but below the anaerobic threshold. Training zones help us to do this, and one of the most recognised methods of calculating these is the **Karvonen principle**. Karvonen suggests a training intensity of between 60% and 75% of maximum heart rate, using the following calculation:

60% = resting heart rate + 0.6 (maximum heart rate − resting heart rate)

75% = resting heart rate + 0.75 (maximum heart rate − resting heart rate)

1.2 Progression

Progression involves the gradual application of overload. It is important to overload the body in order to improve fitness, but this should be done progressively, to avoid illness and to take health issues into account.

1.3 Specificity

The training should be relevant to the sport you are training for. For example, a sprinter will perform strength training on the muscles required for his or her event and will carry out speed training to improve the efficiency of the energy system he or she uses when competing.

1.4 Reversibility

Reversibility is often referred to as 'detraining'. If you stop training, due to injury for example, any adaptations that have been developed as a result of training will deteriorate. It is suggested that aerobic adaptations are lost more quickly than strength adaptations.

1.5 Moderation

Over-training can lead to injury.

1.6 Variance

A training programme needs to have variety in order to maintain interest and motivation.

1.7 Warm-up

A warm-up helps prepare the body for exercise and should always be carried out at the start of any training session. There are three stages:

- **pulse-raising activity** to increase the amount of oxygen being delivered to the muscles
- **stretching/flexibility exercises**, concentrating especially on those joints and muscles that will be most active during the training session
- **performing the movement patterns** that are to be carried out, such as practising shooting in basketball or netball, or dribbling in hockey or football

A warm-up can have the following physiological effects:

- The release of adrenalin increases heart rate and dilates capillaries. This allows more oxygen to be delivered to the skeletal muscles.
- An increase in muscle temperature enables oxygen to dissociate more easily from haemoglobin and allows for an increase in enzyme activity, making energy readily available.
- An increase in muscle temperature causes greater elasticity of the muscle fibres. This leads to an increase in the speed and force of contraction.
- An increase in the speed of nerve impulse conduction makes us more alert.
- Efficient movement at joints occurs through an increased production of synovial fluid.

1.8 Cool-down

It is important to perform a cool-down at the end of any physical activity, as it helps return the body to its pre-exercise state more quickly. A cool-down consists of some form of light exercise to keep heart rate elevated. This keeps blood flow high and allows oxygen to be flushed through the muscles, removing and oxidising any lactic acid that remains. Performing light exercise also allows the skeletal muscle pump to keep working and prevents blood from pooling in the veins.

A cool-down may also result in limiting the effect of **delayed onset of muscle soreness** (DOMS), which is characterised by tender and painful muscles often experienced some 24–48 hours after heavy exercise. This soreness is due to structural damage to muscle fibres and the connective tissue surrounding them. DOMS usually occurs following excessive eccentric contraction, when muscle fibres are put under a lot of strain. This type of muscular contraction occurs mostly from weight training and plyometrics.

2 Types of training

2.1 Continuous training

Continuous training involves exercise without rest intervals and concentrates on developing endurance, thereby placing stress on the aerobic energy system. Examples include exercises such as cycling, jogging and swimming. In order to gain any improvement in aerobic fitness, it is important to apply the principles of training outlined above.

2.2 Fartlek training

Fartlek is a slightly different method of continuous training; the word 'fartlek' means 'speed-play' in Swedish. Here, the performer varies the pace of a run to stress both the aerobic and anaerobic energy systems.

This is a much more demanding type of training and will improve an individual's VO_2 (max) (the maximum volume of oxygen that can be taken in and used in 1 minute) and recovery process. A typical session lasts for approximately 40 minutes, with the intensity ranging from low to high.

2.3 Altitude training

Altitude training is the practice by some endurance athletes of training for several weeks at high altitude. The partial pressure of oxygen drops as altitude increases, usually by up to 50% at an altitude of 5 000 m. This causes a reduction in the diffusion gradient between the air and the lungs, and between the alveoli and the blood. Therefore haemoglobin is not fully saturated, and the blood has less capacity for carrying oxygen. As less oxygen is delivered to working muscles, there is an earlier onset of fatigue, resulting in a decrease in performance of aerobic activities.

The body adapts to a relative lack of oxygen by increasing the concentration of red blood cells and haemoglobin. It is claimed that when athletes who have trained at high altitude participate in competitions at lower altitudes, they still have a higher concentration of red blood cells for 10–14 days, giving them a competitive advantage. A higher concentration of red blood cells allows more oxygen to be supplied to the muscles, resulting in higher performance.

However, altitude training is expensive, and the benefits can be lost quickly on return to sea level. A performer may also suffer from altitude sickness and experience difficulty during initial training sessions, resulting in a detraining effect.

2.4 Interval training

Interval training can be used for both aerobic and anaerobic training. It intersperses periods of work with recovery periods. Four main variables are used to ensure the training is specific:
- duration of the work interval
- intensity or speed of the work interval
- duration of the recovery period
- number of work intervals and recovery periods

It is possible to adapt interval training to overload each of the three energy systems, as summarised in the table below.

Energy system	ATP-PC	Lactic acid	Aerobic
Duration/distance of work interval	60 metres	200 metres	1500 metres
Intensity and duration of work interval	High (10 seconds)	High (35 seconds)	Submaximal
Duration of recovery	30 seconds	110 seconds	5 minutes
Number of work intervals/recovery periods	10	8	3

2.5 Strength training

Some individuals undertake a form of strength training to improve performance in their chosen activity. Improvements in strength result from working against some form of resistance. In this instance, it is important to make any strength-training programme specific to the needs of the activity, and the following factors must be taken into consideration:
- the type of strength to be developed — maximum, elastic or strength endurance
- the muscle groups you wish to improve
- the type of muscle contraction performed in the activity — concentric, eccentric or isometric

Other individuals use strength training for muscle growth. They need to ensure that any exercises they perform will overload the anaerobic energy systems, resulting in hypertrophy of fast-twitch fibres.

Strength can be improved by doing the following types of training:
- weights
- circuits
- pulleys
- plyometrics

2.5a Weights

Weight training is usually described in terms of **sets** and **repetitions**. The number of sets and repetitions you do and the amount of weight you lift depend on the type of strength you wish to improve:
- If maximum strength is the goal, it is necessary to lift high weights with low repetitions.
- If strength endurance is the goal, it is necessary to perform more repetitions of lighter weights.

The choice of exercise should relate to the muscle groups used in the sport — both the agonists and antagonists.

2.5b Circuits

In circuit training, the athlete performs a series of exercises in succession, such as press-ups, sit-ups and squat thrusts. The resistance used is the athlete's body weight, and each successive exercise concentrates on a different muscle group to allow for recovery. A circuit is usually designed for general body conditioning but is easily adapted to meet the needs of an activity.

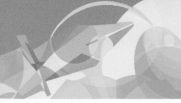

2.5c Pulleys

These are rope or small bungee-type harnesses that allow an athlete to train against resistance. The advantage of this method of strength training is that the exact movement pattern is being performed while the resistance is being applied.

2.5d Plyometrics

Plyometrics is a method of training that improves power or elastic strength. It can be used if leg strength is crucial to successful performance, for example in the long jump and 100 metres sprint in athletics, or rebounding in basketball. It works on the basis that muscles can generate more force if they have previously been stretched. This occurs in plyometrics when, on landing, the muscle performs an eccentric contraction (lengthens under tension) followed immediately by a concentric contraction as the performer jumps up.

2.6 Flexibility training

Sometimes called mobility training, flexibility training involves stretching muscles and connective tissue. A stretch should be held for at least 10 seconds and a session should last for 10 minutes. With regular and repeated stretching, this soft tissue can elongate and this may be beneficial in avoiding injury. There are three main types of flexibility training:
- static stretching
- ballistic stretching
- PNF

2.6a Static stretching

Active stretching occurs when the performer works on one joint, pushing it beyond its point of resistance, lengthening the muscles and connective tissue surrounding it. **Passive stretching** happens when a stretch occurs with the help of an external force, such as a partner, gravity or a wall.

2.6b Ballistic stretching

Ballistic stretching involves performing a stretch with swinging or bouncing movements, to push a body part even further. It is important that this type of stretching is only performed by an individual who is extremely flexible, such as a gymnast or a dancer.

2.6c PNF

PNF stands for **proprioceptive neuromuscular facilitation**, where the muscle is isometrically contracted for a period of at least 10 seconds. It then relaxes and is contracted again, usually going further a second time.

2.7 Planning a training programme

Periodisation is the key to planning a training programme. This involves dividing the year into periods where specific training occurs:
- off-season
- pre-season
- competitive season

This seasonal approach is now commonly adapted to macro-, meso- and microcycles, which describe periods of time that are more prescriptive for individual needs:

- **Macrocycle** — the 'big' period. The performer identifies a macrocycle of about 6–12 months to achieve a long-term goal.
- **Mesocycle** — this describes a short-term goal within the macrocycle, which may last for 6–8 weeks.
- **Microcycle** — this is normally a description of 1 week of training which is repeated throughout the duration of the mesocycle.

2.8 Important factors when planning a specialised training programme

2.8a Thermoregulation

When training and performing, heat is generated in the body as a result of the chemical reactions that take place to produce energy. This heat is then transported to the surface of the skin by the blood, where it is lost through radiation or convection, or through the evaporation of sweat.

During prolonged exercise, or when the body is dehydrated, total blood volume can decrease as more blood is redirected to the skin. This in turn reduces the amount of oxygen available to the working muscles and therefore affects performance. In hot conditions, this situation is exacerbated. It is essential to acclimatise, so that the body can modify the control systems that regulate blood flow to the skin and sweating.

2.8b Respiratory exchange ratio (RER)

Energy sources such as carbohydrates, fats and protein can all be oxidised to produce energy. For a certain volume of oxygen, the energy released will depend upon the energy source. Calculating the RER will determine which of these energy sources is being oxidised. RER is the ratio of carbon dioxide produced to oxygen consumed, and is referred to as the **respiratory quotient** (RQ):

- An RER value between 0.7 and 1.0 = a mix of carbohydrate and fat.
- An RER value of approximately 0.8 = protein.
- An RER value greater than 1.0 = anaerobic respiration, as more carbon dioxide is being produced than oxygen consumed.

Examiner's tip

Make sure you can give the relevant training method for each component of fitness, e.g. aerobic capacity (cardio-respiratory endurance) can be improved by continuous, fartlek and interval training. Exam questions often concern interval training. You may be required to adapt interval training to overload one of the three energy systems.

By the end of this topic, you should be able to:
- define the fitness components and suggest methods of testing for each
- understand aerobic capacity (VO$_2$ max) and describe the limiting factors on performance
- assess the validity and the reliability of fitness tests and understand the principles of maximal and submaximal tests

1 *Physical fitness*

Physical fitness is the ability to perform daily tasks without undue fatigue. It consists of:
- **physical/health components** — aerobic capacity, strength, flexibility, body composition
- **skill/motor components** — speed, balance, reaction time, coordination, agility

Component	Definition	Method of testing	How to improve
Aerobic capacity	Ability to take in and use oxygen	Douglas bag Multi-stage fitness test PWC 170 test	Continuous training
Strength Maximum	Maximum force a muscle can exert in a single voluntary contraction	Hand grip dynamometer	Weight training — high weights, low repetitions
Elastic	Ability to overcome resistance with a high speed of contraction	Wingate test	Plyometrics
Strength endurance	Ability of a muscle to perform repeated contractions and withstand fatigue	NCF abdominal curl	Circuits
Flexibility Static Dynamic	Range of movement round a joint Resistance of a joint to movement	Sit and reach test Goniometer (angle measure)	Static Ballistic PNF
Body composition	Physiological make-up of an individual in terms of the distribution of fat and lean body mass	Skin fold test	Weight training to gain muscle growth Continuous training to lose fat
Speed	How fast a person can move a specified distance or how quickly a body part can be put into motion	30 metre sprint test	Interval training to improve ATP/PC and lactic acid systems
Balance	Ability to keep the centre of mass over the base of support; it can be static, such as a handstand, or dynamic, where balance is retained in motion	Balance board	No specific method of training
Reaction time	Time taken from detection of a stimulus to the initiation of a response	Metre rule test	Sprint starts
Coordination	Ability of the motor and nervous systems to interact	Alternate hand/wall ball test	Skills training
Agility	Ability to move and position the body quickly and effectively while under control	Illinois agility run	Shuttle sprints
Power	Work performed per unit of time: a combination of strength and speed	Vertical jump	Weight training, plyometrics

2 | Aerobic capacity (VO$_2$ (max))

Aerobic capacity is often referred to using different terms such as **stamina**, **VO$_2$ (max)** or **cardiovascular endurance**. In simple terms, aerobic capacity is the ability to take in and use oxygen. This is dependent on three factors:

- how effectively an individual can inspire and expire
- once an individual has inspired, how effective the transportation of the oxygen is from the lungs to where it is needed
- how well that oxygen is then used

Aerobic capacity is important for participation in continuous, submaximal activity, such as jogging or cycling. In an average performer, it is usual to work at around 65 % of VO$_2$ (max). Working harder than this will result in crossing the anaerobic threshold, when the aerobic system is no longer the main energy provider and instead the ATP-PC and lactic acid systems are the predominant methods of re-synthesising ATP. Elite athletes can work at a much higher percentage of their VO$_2$ (max) before crossing the anaerobic threshold (usually 85 %). A person's VO$_2$ (max) is largely genetically determined, although there are differences that occur due to both gender and age.

2.1 Differences in gender

A male long-distance runner will have a VO$_2$ (max) of approximately 70 ml/min/kg, whereas a female long-distance runner will have a VO$_2$ (max) of around 60 ml/min/kg. This is because the average female is smaller than the average male. Females have:

- a smaller left ventricle and therefore a lower stroke volume
- a lower maximum cardiac output
- a lower blood volume, which results in lower haemoglobin levels
- a lower tidal volume and ventilatory volume

2.2 Differences in age

As we get older, our VO$_2$ (max) decreases as our body systems become less efficient:

- maximum heart rate drops by around 5–7 beats per minute per decade
- an increase in peripheral resistance results in a decrease of maximum stroke volume
- blood pressure increases both at rest and during exercise
- less air is exchanged in the lungs due to a decline in vital capacity and an increase in residual air

3 | Validity and reliability of testing

All fitness tests are subject to questions of:

- **validity** — does the test measure exactly what it sets out to? Is the test sport-specific?
- **reliability** — is the test accurate? Can it be repeated?

Factors to take into account when testing include:

- the need for the tester to be experienced
- the need for the equipment to be standardised
- the importance of the sequencing of tests
- the performer's motivation levels
- repetition of tests to avoid human error

4   *General advantages of fitness tests*

- Quick and/or easy testing procedures are involved.
- Little equipment is needed.
- Lots of data are available in order to compare results.
- Predictions are generally accurate.
- Objective data are collected.
- They are time saving (e.g. when testing large groups together).
- The tests are sport-specific and/or muscle-specific.

5   *General limitations of fitness tests*

- Some tests are not sport-specific. They do not replicate specific movements and/or actions.
- Some tests are predictive. They do not use direct measures and can therefore be inaccurate.
- Some tests do not consider the sporting environment or the competitive conditions of the activity.

6   *Maximal and submaximal testing*

Maximal tests, such as the multi-stage fitness test or the Wingate test, require the performer to work to exhaustion. This can be problematic:

- It is difficult to ensure the performer is working to a maximum.
- It depends on how the person feels on the day and the degree of motivation for the test.
- Ethical considerations — forcing a performer to work to his or her maximum can lead to overexertion and injury. It is important to screen an individual before he or she carries out fitness tests (PAR-Q), and to ensure the tests are appropriate to the age, sex and current fitness level of the performer.

Submaximal tests do not require the performer to work to exhaustion and motivation is no longer an issue. However, these tests rely on estimating or predicting, and are therefore not completely objective. This can cause problems in terms of validity and reliability.

Examiner's tip

Make sure you learn the table on page 53 comprehensively, as previous questions have asked for definitions of components, how they are tested and how they can be improved. Try to relate fitness components to specific sports performers. Look further than just an explanation of the fitness test: is it maximal or submaximal? Is it valid and/or reliable for the sport in question?

By the end of this topic, you should be able to describe and explain the physiological adaptations that take place after a prolonged period of:

- aerobic training
- strength training
- flexibility training

Physiological adaptations are long-lasting changes that occur in the body as a result of following a training programme. These changes take place to allow improvement in fitness. The type of training you choose to do will result in specific adaptations.

1 Adaptations to aerobic training

If you perform continuous, fartlek or aerobic interval training over a period of time, physiological adaptations take place that would make the initial training sessions appear easy. This is because your aerobic capacity/VO_2 (max) improves as the adaptations outlined in the table below take place.

Heart	Hypertrophy of the myocardium (heart gets bigger and stronger)	Increase in stroke volume and maximum cardiac output	Decrease in resting heart rate	
Lungs	Maximum minute ventilation increases	Respiratory muscles become more efficient	Increase in resting lung volume	Diffusion rates improve
Blood	Blood volume increases, due mainly to an increase in blood plasma and a small increase in red blood cells		Blood less acidic at rest but more acidic during exercise due to a greater tolerance of lactic acid	
Vascular system	Aerobic training can increase the elasticity of the arterial walls, making it easier to cope with fluctuations in blood pressure		Increase in the density of the capillary networks surrounding the lungs and skeletal muscle	
Muscles	Increase in myoglobin	Increase in mitochondria	Increase in activity of the respiratory enzymes	Increase in energy stores in the muscle cell (glycogen and triglycerides)

2 Adaptations to strength training

The type of strength training you do will result in specific adaptations. With weight training, for example, light weights and high repetitions allow adaptations to occur in slow oxidative fibres, whereas heavy weights and low repetitions allow adaptations in fast glycolytic fibres.

2.1 Aerobic adaptations in slow oxidative fibres

- hypertrophy of slow-twitch fibres
- increase in mitochondria and myoglobin
- increase in glycogen and triglyceride stores
- increase in capillaries

2.2 Anaerobic adaptations to fast-twitch fibres

- hypertrophy of fast oxidative glycolytic and fast glycolytic fibres
- increase in ATP and PC stores
- increase in glycogen stores
- greater tolerance of lactic acid

2.3 Neural adaptations to strength training

- More strength can be generated by the recruitment of more motor units.
- The inhibitory effect of the golgi tendon organs is reduced, which allows the muscle to stretch further and generate more force.

3   *Physiological adaptations to flexibility training*

Adaptations occur after a period of flexibility training. The tendons, ligaments and muscles surrounding a joint have elastic properties, which allow a change in length. There is more of a change to muscle tissue than to tendons or ligaments.

Examiner's tip

Look at the exam question and work out if it asks for aerobic or anaerobic adaptations, or for both. The next stage is to assess which specific adaptations are required; for example, if the question asks for cardiovascular adaptations, you need to talk about the heart *and* the blood.

By the end of this topic, you should:
● be aware of both legal and illegal ergogenic aids
● understand the positive and negative effects ergogenic aids can have on performance, and any side effects
● be able to identify the types of performer who would benefit from the use of each aid

All athletes want to improve their performance, and there are both legal and illegal methods of achieving this (in addition to training). Substances that improve performance are referred to as **ergogenic aids**.

Method of enhancement	Description of method	Reasons why this method is used	Side effects
High carbo-hydrate diet (legal)	A diet high in carbo-hydrates such as pasta, rice and bread will increase glycogen levels	Compensates for lower levels of glycogen during exercise	None
Glycogen loading (legal)	This takes place 6 days before an important competition: for the first 3 days, training on a high fat and protein diet occurs; on the last 3 days there is light training on a high carbohydrate diet	Can increase glycogen levels and therefore increase endurance performance	More water can be stored in the muscle, but such an extreme change in routine can cause slight physiolog-ical problems
Amphetamines (illegal)	Stimulants	Decrease tiredness, increase metabolism; individual is more alert	Insomnia, weight loss, cardiovascular problems that can lead to death
Blood doping (illegal)	Blood is removed and stored; the body then compensates for this loss and makes more red blood cells; the stored blood is then injected back into the performer, giving a higher red blood cell count	Improves aerobic capacity through increasing the oxygen-carrying capacity of the body, allowing the performer to work for longer	The viscosity of the blood can increase, leading to clotting and a risk of death
Anabolic steroids (illegal)	Artificially produced hormones	Promote muscle growth and lean body weight	Liver damage, acne, excessive aggression
Caffeine (legal)	Stimulant	Thought to improve the mobilisation of fatty acids in the body	Increased danger of dehydration
Beta-blockers (illegal)	Help to calm the individual down	Can improve accuracy in precision sports through steadying the nerves	Tiredness due to low blood pressure and slower heart rate
Creatine monohydrate (legal)	A supplement used to increase the amount of phosphocreatine stored in the muscles	Allows the ATP-PC system to last longer and can help improve recovery times	No harmful side effects known

Method of enhancement	Description of method	Reasons why this method is used	Side effects
EPO (illegal)	A natural hormone produced by the kidneys to increase red blood cells; it can now be artificially manufactured to cause an increase in haemoglobin levels	An increase in the oxygen-carrying capacity of the body can lead to an increase in the amount of work performed	Can result in blood clotting, stroke and, in a few cases, death
Human growth hormone (illegal)	Hormones	Increases muscle mass and causes a decrease in fat	Heart and nerve diseases, glucose intolerance, high levels of blood fats
Protein supplements (legal)	Amino acids	Enhance muscle repair and growth	Excess stress placed on the kidneys
Herbal remedies, such as ginseng (legal)	Natural product taken as part of a diet	Thought to enhance muscle recovery	Diarrhoea, skin rashes, nervousness, hypertension, sleeplessness
Gene therapy (illegal)	Synthetic gene	Lasts for a long period of time; can produce large amounts of naturally occurring muscle-building hormones; hard to detect as they do not enter the bloodstream	Depending on the gene, problems with the heart and liver; may cause death

Examiner's tip

Questions often require candidates to select a relevant ergogenic aid and explain its effect on performance and its possible side effects. Be sure to consider the needs of the performer before selecting an aid to discuss. If the question asks you to consider an endurance athlete, for example, then steroids are not the relevant aid.

Section 2
Skills acquisition & sports psychology

1 Skill and ability

By the end of this topic, you should:
- know the different characteristics of skill and ability
- understand the relationship between skill and ability
- be able to classify skills

1 Characteristics of skill and ability

1.1 Skills

Skilful movement in sport can be identified using the following features:
- A skill is **learned**, usually as a result of some form of practice.
- Skill is **aesthetic** or pleasing to look at — it is **fluent**, **controlled** and **smooth**.
- A skill is a **goal-directed** movement when the performer has some kind of achievement in mind, such as a delicate chip from the edge of the green in golf to get the ball as close to the target as possible.
- A skill is performed with **economical** use of energy — it is **efficient**.
- A skill is **consistent** — for example, a good goal kicker in a rugby game always gets the ball between the posts.

A useful revision technique to help you recall factual information is to use a memorable phrase or rhyme. For example, you might use the phrase 'Lucky cats get a fish consistently every Saturday evening'. This will help you to remember the characteristics of skill as follows:
- **l**ucky — **l**earned
- **c**ats — **c**ontrolled
- **g**et — **g**oal-directed
- **a** — **a**esthetic
- **f**ish — **f**luent
- **c**onsistently — **c**onsistent
- **e**very — **e**fficient
- **S**aturday — **s**mooth
- **e**vening — **e**conomical

1.2 Ability

Ability in sport is an innate characteristic required for performing movement. We might be born with good coordination, for example, which could help us to develop passing skills after periods of practice. Abilities are therefore said to be the building blocks of skill; they last a long time and can be developed or enhanced by our early experiences.

Other definitions with which you should be familiar are:
- **perceptual ability** — the ability to sense and interpret information, such as the midfield player in hockey assessing the field before making a pass
- **gross motor ability** — the characteristic required for large muscle group movements, such as the strength needed for a tackle in rugby

The relationship between skill and ability is summarised in Figure 26. The diagram shows that people are born with specific abilities that can be improved by early coaching and childhood play and through access to good facilities. For example, a parent who takes a young child to a gymnastics club helps to lay a foundation for future skills development. A variety of practice and early games also enhances abilities.

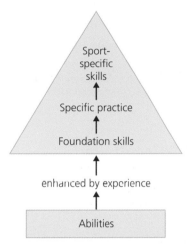

Figure 26

Once abilities have been enhanced, they can develop into **foundation skills** such as throwing, catching, kicking, evading, balancing and jumping. Only after a period of **specific practice** will the inherent abilities develop into **sport-specific skills**. A netball player uses the abilities of coordination and manual dexterity to develop the foundation skills of throwing and catching before the specific netball pass can be developed.

Abilities are specific to the skills they underpin. There is no such thing as general ability, but rather a number of abilities that can be used in the learning of specific sport skills. Natural speed, power and coordination are a starting point from which to coach a 100 m-sprint start. Other abilities that are present in a sports performer include **strength**, **flexibility**, **stamina**, **static balance**, **agility** and **visual acuity**.

2 *Skill classification*

Attempts to classify skills can help sports coaches to plan and prepare their coaching sessions. Skills are usually classified on a sliding scale called a **skills continuum**, which shows the range or extent to which a skill meets certain criteria. The continuum can also reveal how a skill differs depending on the situation. The criteria used to classify skills are as follows:

- open/closed
- discrete/serial/continuous
- self-paced/externally paced
- gross/fine
- complex/simple
- low-organised/highly organised

2.1 Open/closed

An **open skill** is affected by the sporting environment. It can be changed or adapted by the performer, and some decision-making is required. An example is a rugby pass, when the ball carrier decides which player to pass to, or a tennis return, which may depend on the opponent's shot. On the other hand, a **closed skill** involves less decision making;

it can become a habit and tends not to be affected by the environment. An example is a shot put performed repeatedly in the same throwing circle.

An environmental decisions continuum would look like Figure 27. Note how the football pass and the tennis return are both open skills, but one is thought to be more open than the other. The continuum shows the range between skills.

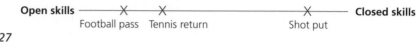

Figure 27

2.2 Discrete/serial/continuous

A **discrete skill** has a short time-span with a clear beginning and end, for example a tennis serve. A **continuous skill** has no clear beginning or end — the end of one part of the movement links into the next, such as the leg movement required when cycling. A **serial skill** is a set of discrete movements, linked together in a necessary order to form a more continuous task. An example is the leap, jump and kick which might be linked together to form a dance routine.

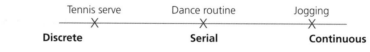

Figure 28

2.3 Self-paced/externally paced

A **self-paced skill** is where the performer can decide how to execute the (usually closed) skill and control the rate of execution. For example, when a penalty is taken in football the player can decide to place the ball in the corner of the goal or 'blast' it past the keeper. An **externally paced skill** is one during which the rate of execution is outside the control of the performer, who may have to react to external conditions. It is usually an open skill. In sailing, for instance, the speed of the wind dictates the pace of the boat.

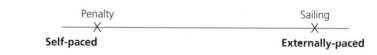

Figure 29

2.4 Gross/fine

A **fine skill** has small, delicate muscle movements, such as the finger control required in a pistol shot at a target. A **gross skill** uses large muscle group movements, such as the movement of the biceps and triceps during a badminton drop shot. Most skills in sport are gross skills.

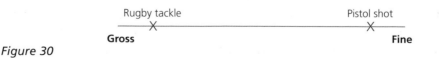

Figure 30

2.5 Complex/simple

A **complex skill** involves a high level of decision making and has a large cognitive or 'thinking' element. A passing sequence in netball or a set of six tackles in rugby league are examples. A **simple skill**, such as a forward roll in gymnastics, has a limited amount of information to process and a smaller cognitive element.

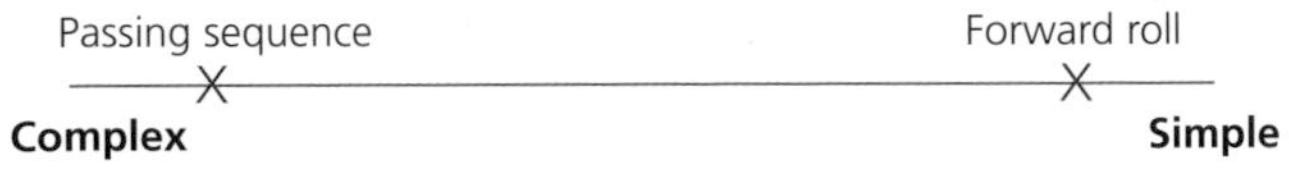

Passing sequence   Forward roll
       X   X
Complex   **Simple**

Figure 31

2.6 Low-organised/highly organised

A **low-organised skill** can be broken down into its parts, or sub-routines, quite easily. When teaching a swimming stroke, the coach can teach the arm and leg actions separately using a float. A **highly organised skill** is hard to break down because it is fast and ballistic in its execution, for example a golf swing.

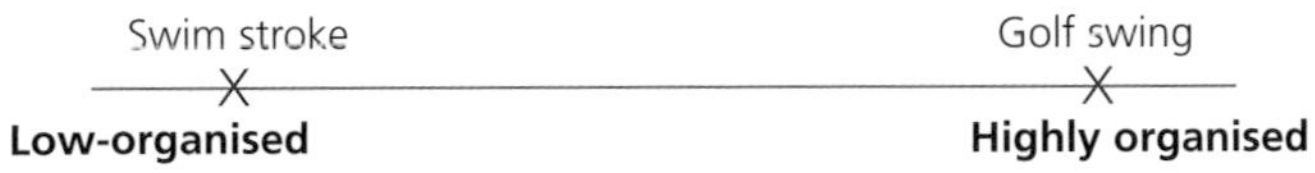

Swim stroke   Golf swing
       X   X
Low-organised   **Highly organised**

Figure 32

2.7 Using skill classification

An awareness of skill classification is important for sports coaches, who must consider the type of skill when planning practices and training sessions.

If the skill is open, a coach should vary practice because environmental conditions change. He or she could manipulate the environment to make practice more like the real game situation by setting up drills that require the performer to adapt to attacking and defending. Performance will then improve, because the player's ability to think and interpret information should be developed and the selective attention process made faster, allowing the player more time to concentrate on the task. The player may even learn to anticipate by picking up environmental signals quickly and experiencing different situations within the game.

A closed skill can be practised by repeating the same movement, as environmental conditions stay the same. This allows the skill to be learned quickly and the performance can be 'grooved' into a habitual response. Performers control the rate of execution, so they need to gain experience of doing the skill at their own pace. This allows attention to detail and the development of a feel for the whole task, with improved **kinaesthesis** or inner sense of the required movement.

Should the coach want to improve a player's fitness, practice without rest intervals or **massed practice** may be used. Massed practice is used for discrete or simple skills and allows a feel for the skill to be developed quickly. It could therefore be beneficial for a beginner in the early stages of learning. Should the players need a rest (especially beginners), **distributed practice** could be used. Distributed practice is used for complex or serial skills and allows the pace of learning to be more controlled and any fatigue to be avoided. The coach could use the rest interval to improve performance further by giving feedback and allowing time for the players to think about the requirements of the task.

Examiner's tip

Exam questions on abilities and skills often require the candidate to name three characteristics of skill or ability. Make sure that you name three *different* characteristics. For a skill, the terms 'goal-directed', 'consistent' and 'learned' would get the marks, but 'smooth', 'fluent' and 'efficient' might be considered too similar to gain separate marks.

When you answer questions on skill classification, be careful not to fall into the trap of describing a skill instead of explaining why it is classified as it is. For example, a football pass is open because the sporting environment influences it and decisions are needed, not because you have to kick the ball to another player.

The AQA and OCR exam boards cover skills and psychology in similar ways. However, the Edexcel specification does not cover skills acquisition in as much detail.

By the end of this topic, you should understand:
- the methods used by sports performers to select and utilise information from the environment
- how a performer stores important information from the environment
- how information is collected and organised by the performer

1 *Stages of information processing*

Figure 33 explains the four basic stages of information processing.

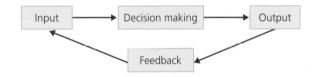

Figure 33

The first stage, the **sensory input**, involves selecting relevant information from the surroundings. This information forms the basis of a **decision-making** process in stage two, when the **response** is selected, and then initiated in stage three. After the response, **feedback** can be used to amend any incorrect movements.

To understand the concepts of information processing fully, a more detailed approach is necessary. The models of Welford and Whiting, shown in Figures 34 and 35, illustrate the main features. Each part of the models should be considered in turn.

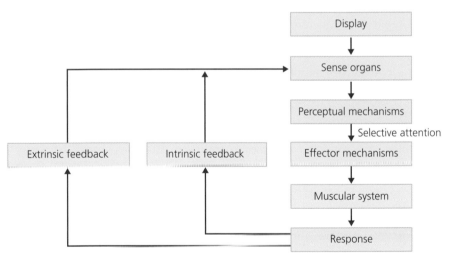

Figure 34 The Welford model

The **display** is the sporting environment from which information is selected. It includes a wealth of detail, such as the court, umpire, crowd and opposition in tennis. The **sense organs** are responsible for picking up the required information from the display in the form of the **receptors**, namely **vision** (seeing the flight of the ball), **audition** (hearing the sound of the ball hit the racket) and the sensors within the body called the **propriocep-tors**. These help to provide the sense of **balance** or equilibrium (such as the balance of the feet when preparing to receive serve), the sense of **touch** (such as the feel of the racket in the hand), and the sense of **kinaesthesis** (the inner feeling of tension within the muscles and joints). When serving in tennis, for example, kinaesthesis informs us that the arm is raised without the need to look.

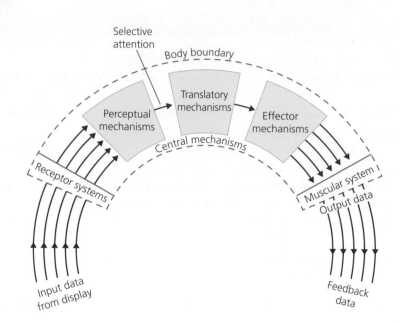

Figure 35 The Whiting model

A decision on the appropriate response is made in the **perceptual mechanisms**. However, before a decision can be made, the wealth of information picked up by the receptors has to be filtered and coded, otherwise there would simply be too much information for the brain to cope with.

A process called **selective attention** is responsible for separating the **stimulus** (relevant and important information) from the **noise** (irrelevant information). It is the stimulus (e.g. the ball in tennis) that is acted upon, while the noise (e.g. the crowd of spectators) is disregarded. Selective attention allows the performer to concentrate and focus on the correct stimulus, and avoids an overload of information.

In the **translatory mechanisms**, a feature unique to the Whiting model, the relevant information is compared to the memory system in an attempt to recognise the stimulus, and a decision on the correct response is made. Impulses are then sent to the working muscles via a network of nerves called the **effector mechanisms**. On receiving an impulse, the muscles required to perform the movement begin to contract and a **response**, such as the tennis return, can take place. As this response is being performed, various forms of **feedback** can be used to detect and correct errors in the movement.

The whole sequence of information processing can occur in fractions of a second; skilled performers are able to process information quickly, being particularly good at selecting relevant information from the display.

2 *Feedback*

Feedback is information acquired during and after the response and is used to aid movement correction. It improves performance because it either tells performers what they are doing wrong or gives reinforcement for correct actions so that they become habitual. Feedback also provides performers with motivation and confidence.

The performer can obtain feedback in various ways:
● **Extrinsic feedback** comes from an outside source, such as a coach telling performers why they missed a shot.

- **Intrinsic feedback** comes from within and could be the sense of kinaesthesis informing performers why they missed the shot.
- **Positive feedback** is a motivator and tells the performers what they got right. It is useful for beginners, and may come in the form of praise from the coach.
- **Negative feedback** is about error correction and the fine-tuning technique used by experts.
- **Knowledge of results** is a starting point for beginners — it is about success or failure. Did the basketball shot go into the ring or not?
- **Knowledge of performance** is appropriate for a more advanced player and concerns improvements in technique. Why did the ball go in the ring?
- **Terminal feedback** might come about after the game and could include the coach's summary of the performance.
- **Concurrent feedback** may come during the game and could be an internal summary of the strengths of the opponent.

Different types of feedback can occur at the same time. After a game, a coach's summary of a performance could be external, terminal and negative. The types of feedback appropriate for a novice are:
- extrinsic, since he or she needs help from the coach when performing
- positive, since encouragement is needed
- knowledge of results to help as a starting point

For an expert performer, intrinsic feedback can be used along with negative feedback and knowledge of performance, to help in error correction and improve technique.

For feedback to be as effective as possible, it should be given immediately after the game. It should be specific and relevant so that the player can remember it. It is a good idea to set a target for the player to help improvement. For example, a rugby player who has received external feedback on tackling technique from the coach could be set a target of making five more tackles per game. Any feedback should be given in clear, concise terms so that the performer is not confused.

3 The memory system

Memory is defined as the storage of the results of information processing activity. It can be illustrated in a flow diagram, such as Figure 36.

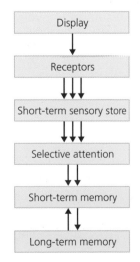

Figure 36

Information picked up from the display by the receptors is held immediately for a fraction of a second in the short-term sensory store, a temporary and transient holding space. By using selective attention, this store begins to filter and code the information into stimulus and noise. The stimulus is then passed on to the **short-term memory**, which begins to work on it and help the performer in decision-making by operating in tandem with the **long-term memory**. Stored images can be retrieved from the long-term memory for current use, and practised images can be moved from the short-term memory to the long-term memory for storage. The short-term memory has a limited capacity and can only process around seven items of information — hence the importance of selective attention.

The short-term memory is called the **working memory** because it has responsibility for the present action and has a link to both the sensory store, from which it receives the stimulus, and the long-term memory, from which it can retrieve information that has been encountered in the past and stored. The long-term memory is a large storage system in which the images of skills and practices from sport have been filed away, rather like the data files in a computer, in a logical sequence called a **motor programme**.

The long-term memory has a large capacity, and the information stored in it can last a lifetime. Once you have learned to swim, you never forget, even if your technique becomes a little rusty.

3.1 Storage of information

When information is stored in the long-term memory, it is said to be 'coded'. Information can be coded more easily by:
- **repetition**
- the **presentation of a clear image**
- an **intense stimulus** that could be pleasurable or painful (e.g. as a sports performer, you might have a clear recollection of a time when you were injured)

A coach might help to promote effective storage of skills by constantly instructing performers, by giving a clear demonstration of the skill, perhaps involving a role model or expert, and by conducting a pleasurable or intense training session.

Other ways to ensure that skills are stored in the long-term memory include:
- **associating the image of a skill you are learning with one you already know**, particularly if the two skills are similar, e.g. you might use your knowledge of an overhead tennis serve to help you to store the image of a volleyball serve
- **mental rehearsal**, when the image of a skill is repeated in the mind without movement
- **rewarding and reinforcing good performances**, perhaps by saying 'well done' after a good shot

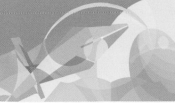

Examiner's tip

Questions on information processing often relate to one of the information-processing models. A useful approach is to draw the model or use the diagram of the model you are given and to explain each part in sequential order, using an example at each stage. As a starting point, you might state that information is picked up from the display, which is the sporting environment — for example, the net, ball, crowd, umpire and opponent in tennis.

Feedback is often referred to in the exam as an aid to performance and you are required to state its benefits, which include:

● building confidence
● providing motivation
● correcting errors

Any types of feedback should be demonstrated with an example, such as extrinsic feedback being the coach telling the swimmer why a turn was so effective.

Questions on the memory system may require you to name some of the features of the various storage parts of the memory. For example, you might state that the long-term memory is said to have a limitless capacity, to last a lifetime and to store motor programmes. Make sure that you read the question carefully, and do not confuse the short-term sensory store with the short-term memory.

By the end of this topic, you should:
● be able to define reaction, movement and response time
● know all the factors affecting response time
● know how to develop faster reaction times in sports performers

1 *Reaction, movement and response*

Reaction time measures a performer's ability to sense and interpret information before making a movement in sport, based on perceptual ability. The relationship between reaction time, movement time and response time for an athletics race is illustrated in Figure 37.

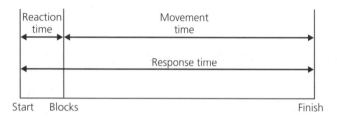

Figure 37

This shows us that reaction time is the time between the onset of the stimulus and the onset of the response. There is no movement in reaction time; it is the processing of the stimulus before movement takes place. For example, at the start of the race, the reaction time is the period from hearing the gun until just prior to leaving the blocks.

Movement time is the time from the beginning to the completion of the task, so that in our example it would be from the first movement until hitting the tape at the finish.

Response time is from the onset of the stimulus to the completion of the task, which in our example is the time from hearing the gun until hitting the tape.

Response time is therefore the sum of reaction time and movement time.

In sport, the more choices the performer has to make, the slower the response time will be. A **simple reaction time** is when a performer needs to react to just one stimulus, such as the gun at the start of a 100 m race; with a focused approach, the reaction time should be quick.

A **choice reaction time** is when a performer has to choose from a number of options, such as a midfield player in football deciding which player to pass to. Reaction time in this example would be slower.

The relationship between reaction time and the number of choices is explained by **Hicks's law**, which states that an increase from a simple reaction time of one choice to a choice reaction time of three or four choices would cause a relatively large increase in reaction time. However, an increase in the number of choices from four to five, six or seven would only increase reaction time by a relatively small amount. Hicks's law is illustrated in Figure 38.

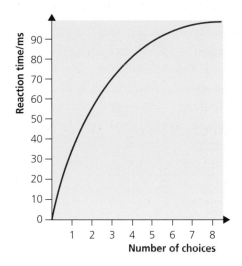

Figure 38

2 Influences on reaction time and response time

Reaction time is influenced by the following factors (which in turn affects response time, since it includes both reaction time and movement time):

- **Age** affects response time, as older performers tend to react more slowly. A veteran in a sprint race would not be as quick off the blocks as a young athlete.
- **Experienced** players tend to react more quickly because they can anticipate more readily. In a squash game, the experienced player dominates the centre of the court, knowing where the ball will land, while the less experienced player is forced to run around the court.
- Some studies have shown that men react faster than women, so **gender** might affect reaction time.
- The effect of performance-enhancing **drugs** might affect reaction time, so that an athlete taking steroids might start faster in a swimming race.
- The level of **fitness** affects reaction time, so that an athlete who has undergone strength and power training might produce a faster start.
- We tend to react more quickly to an **intense stimulus**, such as a loud shout from a team mate in football.

3 Improving response time

Coaches use their knowledge of response time to develop fast reactions in their players.

The strategies used to improve reaction time include:

- mental rehearsal (running through a performance in the mind without movement)
- getting the performer to focus (e.g. an athlete concentrating on a point down the track before the start of a race)
- enhancing the fitness levels of the performer

Fast reactions are also promoted by the ability to anticipate. There are three types of anticipation:

- **effector anticipation** — getting a feel for the skill, rather like a cricketer would get a feel for the wicket before anticipating the pitch of the ball
- **receptor anticipation** — experienced players are good at anticipation because they can read a game by looking at the stance and body language of their opponent, i.e. using the cues, or stimuli, from the environment (using receptor systems)
- **perceptual anticipation** — developed from external sources, such as by studying an opponent on video or receiving extrinsic feedback from a coach on an opponent's style of play

Anticipation in sport is seen as a gamble: if you anticipate correctly, your reaction times will be quick; however, incorrect anticipation can cause reaction times to be slow.

There are other influences on reaction time that are worthy of special note. The **single-channel hypothesis** attempts to explain why we are slower if we have to process more than one stimulus. It states that each stimulus we process has to progress through a single track, so that a subsequent stimulus must wait for the one before it to be processed before it can be dealt with, rather like a queue of cars waiting at a road junction. This is illustrated in Figure 39.

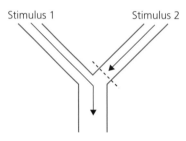

Figure 39

The **psychological refractory period** (PRP) is a moment in time when we are forced to 'freeze', due to the presentation of two stimuli in close succession. Like the single-channel hypothesis, this theory seeks to explain why a delay is caused when we have to process more than one stimulus. The PRP means that when a second stimulus arrives before the response to the first stimulus has been processed completely, an inevitable delay will occur because we can only process one stimulus at a time. In tennis, for example, we may be ready to return a passing shot with a forehand volley, but before we can play the shot the ball hits the net and deflects to our backhand side. There will be an inevitable delay: we have to deal with the stimulus affecting the volley, even though we don't play it, before we can deal with the stimulus affecting the backhand. It therefore affects our information processing ability.

Some sports players use their knowledge of the PRP to their advantage by trying to fool their opponent, perhaps by giving a dummy pass in rugby, or by looking one way and passing the other in netball. The PRP is illustrated in Figure 40.

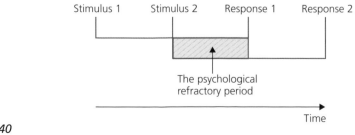

Figure 40

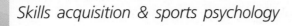

Examiner's tip

A sound knowledge of the definitions of reaction time, movement time and response time, together with sporting examples, will often gain easy marks. Include a diagram to show the relationship between these three definitions if you are not given a diagram to interpret in the question. You should be aware of sporting examples to help you describe the factors that affect response time. Explanations of both the PRP and the single-channel hypothesis are based on the fact that we can only process one stimulus at a time, and you can relate these concepts to each other in any answer.

By the end of this topic, you should:
- understand the benefits of motor programmes for top-level performance
- know how such motor programmes are formed
- be able to explain how less experienced performers control movement using feedback

1 *Motor programmes*

A motor programme is a set of movements, stored in the long-term memory, which specify the components of a skill. It is formed by specific and continued practice, during which internal and external feedback help to check errors and amend performance. Over time, the incorrect and negative aspects of performance are eliminated and the performer is left with a vision of how to carry out the skill perfectly. For example, a novice learning to hit a tennis return concentrates first on getting the ball over the net and into the court and uses internal feedback to sense that a ball that failed to get over the net has been hit too softly. External feedback from the coach would improve early technique and then, once the basis of the shot has been mastered, a period of lengthy practice would perfect the image of the skill and associate it with the accompanying stimulus. The use of mental rehearsal can also help to develop the motor programme.

Once the motor programme is developed, the performance is smooth and efficient, and the information processing aspect of the task is quicker because just one stimulus can trigger the image of the skill. Reaction times are therefore fast and the performer can concentrate on detailed aspects of the skill using the spare attention capacity. Skills can therefore be automatic and habitual in their execution.

1.1 Open-loop control

When the motor programme is developed, it can control the movement of the skill at the highest level of performance. Since feedback has been used to perfect the motor programme, the skill can now be controlled using little conscious feedback, a concept known as **open-loop control**. This is illustrated in Figure 41.

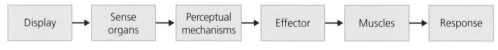

Figure 41

Information is picked up by the receptor systems and filtered by selective attention, so that the stimulus is referred to the memory for decision-making. A message is then sent by the effector mechanism to start the response using muscular contraction. During open-loop control, this process is quick and movement is controlled almost automatically.

Open-loop control can be used in two situations:
- when a closed skill is being performed and a developed motor programme means that there is no need to use feedback; the skill is always performed in the same way
- when the skill is so fast in its execution that there is no time to use feedback (e.g. in tennis, the first serve takes a fraction of a second and there is no time to use feedback during the task, although feedback can be used after the skill has been completed to amend the second serve)

An effective motor programme is stored in the memory logically. The image of the main task is accompanied by the sub-routines or parts of the skill. For example, a throw would be stored in the order shown in Figure 42.

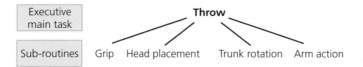

Figure 42

Basic motor programmes, learned as foundation skills, can then be enhanced into more complex, sports-specific skills by continued refining of the performance with feedback from both the coach and from within the performer. The basic throwing action can therefore develop into the sports-specific skill of the netball pass, as shown in Figure 43.

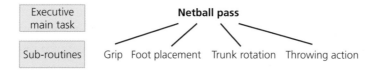

Figure 43

1.2 Closed-loop control

Closed-loop control can be described as an internal self-checking mechanism, used to improve performance. It is illustrated in Figure 44.

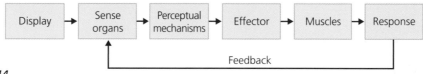

Figure 44

Information is picked up by the receptors and coded using selective attention. A decision on the response is made and sent to the muscles for action using the effector mechanism. As the response is in progress, internal senses associated with kinaesthesis check the movements and detect any errors, which are then corrected. Additional feedback from the coach could also be used to amend future performance. A gymnast on the balance beam would check each step forward and use kinaesthesis to make sure balance was stable before making progress. Any errors would be corrected before the next step was made.

Closed-loop control operates at two levels of competence. If open-loop control operates at level 1, closed-loop control operates at levels 2 and 3. At both levels, feedback is used to check and amend performance:

● At level 2, feedback is used as the task is being performed, usually during more continuous skills. Even advanced performers can use intrinsic feedback to check their movements as they are in action. A downhill skier could check and amend an overbalance as he or she makes progress down the slope, and any adjustments in body position could be made quickly as needed. The current movements may well be compared to a trace held in the memory, and any deviation from this trace would be dealt with.

- At level 3, feedback is again used to check and amend performance. However, because the performer at this level is more likely to be a novice, the process of comparing movements with the memory trace takes longer, and any adjustments in performance are sent through the brain and thought about. Movement may appear to lack fine control at this level, and even extrinsic feedback can be used to help adjust movements.

Examiner's tip

Make sure you can differentiate between the benefits of a motor programme in terms of the efficiency and quick reactions it can produce, and the ways in which it is developed through feedback and practice. You could be asked to name some sub-routines of a skill and to explain how a basic motor programme can become more complex by fine-tuning the performance with specific practice. Closed-loop control requires an example from sport to help you explain how errors are detected and amended by feedback. The gymnastics example in the text above is an appropriate one to use. Remember to include a diagram with your answer and don't forget that the first part of any type of motor control involves decision-making and then the sending of an impulse by the effector mechanism to start muscular contraction.

5 Theories of learning

By the end of this topic, you should:
- understand the theoretical concepts that help skills to be learned in sport
- be able to apply strategies that would be used to promote learning

1 Phases of learning

It has been suggested by sports psychologists Fitts and Posner (1967) that there are three phases of learning, progressing from the beginner stage to the expert stage of performance. The features of each of these phases are given below.

(1) **Cognitive phase:** the performer is a beginner and uses closed-loop control, with a heavy dependence on feedback. Movement is uncoordinated and there are breaks in performance as the player tries to understand the parts of the skill during a trial-and-error session of practice. An example of the cognitive phase in sport is a rugby player watching a demonstration of a drop kick and then trying to copy it.

(2) **Associative phase:** so-named because performers try to compare or associate their current level of performance with that of an expert. The performer tries to eradicate deficiencies with a lengthy period of practice and may again use trial and error to concentrate on improving weaknesses. Both internal feedback and external feedback are used to improve performance. An example of the associative phase would be a rugby player practising the drop kick with the coach and eliminating errors. Motor programmes start to form in this stage.

(3) **Autonomous phase:** by practising continually, the performer has by now developed a motor programme, which is used to control movement. The performer can use spare attention capacity to concentrate on detail, as the motor programme may only require one stimulus to initiate a response. Movement is smooth and fluent. An example of the autonomous phase is an expert rugby player repeating drop kicks with precision to maintain a high level of skill. To remain in the final phase of learning, a performer must sometimes refer back to the associative phase to eliminate any sudden changes in the skill environment, such as a gust of wind that could blow a floating ball off course. Intense practice must continue, and the player may use mental rehearsal to go over the finer points of the performance before a game.

There are various theories and concepts that help the player move up from the cognitive to the autonomous phase of learning. These are addressed below.

2 Observational learning

In sport, we can learn skills by observing and then imitating the demonstrations given to us by coaches, teachers or experts. In order for the demonstration to be successful, the coach might consider four processes that were suggested by Bandura in his model of observational learning:

- First, it is necessary to gain the **attention** of the performer by making the demonstration stand out, perhaps by explaining the relevance, purpose and importance of the skill being shown. A role model or expert could be used to make the demonstration appealing and proficient.
- The second process is to make sure the performer **retains** the demonstration. This might be done by breaking down the skill and giving an accurate and clear presentation of each part, so that the memory system can absorb the necessary information. The skill can be remembered if it is repeated or practised mentally.

- The third process is to enable the performer to **reproduce** the skill being shown by starting with a basic demonstration that is within his or her capability to make sure success is achieved.
- The final process is to **motivate** the player to perform the demonstrated skill by offering positive reinforcement, praise or rewards as success is achieved.

These processes are illustrated in Figure 45.

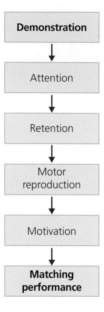

Figure 45

It is more likely that a demonstration will be copied if:
- it is powerful
- it is always accurate
- praise or rewards are offered to the performer
- it is performed by someone of a similar age and gender to the performer — a role model from a similar peer group may make the task seem more achievable

3 Operant conditioning and the stimulus–response (S–R) bond

In sport, we learn by associating the correct response with a stimulus. The theory of operant conditioning explains how correct responses to a stimulus can be made stronger if the action is reinforced and the coach manipulates the performer during and after the performance.

Operant conditioning attempts to shape behaviour and works on the principle that repeated actions are made stronger. It is based on the concept of trial-and-error learning, during which the performer attempts a skill and correct actions are then reinforced by using praise or rewards (**positive reinforcement**). The coach may set easy targets at first to ensure success, and this offers an incentive to continue.

Incorrect actions can be weakened so that they are eliminated. This is done through the use of **negative reinforcement** — withdrawing the praise offered for the correct response — or **punishment**, such as extra training, for an incorrect response.

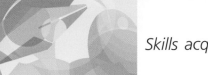

Thorndike suggested three laws to link the stimulus to the response and promote learning:

- The law of **exercise** states that practice will strengthen the S–R bond.
- The law of **effect** states that an **annoyer**, such as criticism, will weaken incorrect actions and that a **satisfier**, such as praise, will strengthen correct actions.
- The law of **readiness** states that the performer must be **capable** of performing the required task — targets must be within the performer's capabilities.

Trial-and-error learning is summarised in Figure 46.

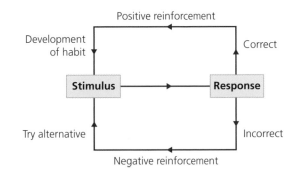

Figure 46

An example of operant conditioning would be a coach encouraging a novice tennis player to perfect a return using trial-and-error practice, offering praise for a good shot and saying nothing for a bad shot. If the player has difficulty, the coach should allow him or her to move closer to the net and then point out the correct hitting action, while criticising the incorrect shot.

4 Cognitive theory of learning

The cognitive theory of learning suggests that a problem-solving approach can help us to learn. Specifically, it helps performers to understand their actions by personally identifying solutions to problems; this is frequently more effective than receiving instruction from another person. It is therefore often referred to as **insight learning**.

When players are presented with a problem, such as how to move an opponent around court when playing badminton, they work out the solution independently. In this case, the tactic might be to play a drop shot and then a long shot. The performers may use past experience to help work out the solution and the problem may be best solved by working on the task as a whole rather than in parts. If the solution is right, they might be motivated to repeat the same response when confronted by a similar problem in the future, especially if they understand why they did it.

5 Transfer of training

The theory of transfer explains why we can take skills from one sport and attempt to use them in another. For example, a netball player might use knowledge of a netball pass to make a pass in basketball. Such transfer of skills can be positive when the knowledge of one skill helps the learning of another, or negative when the knowledge becomes a hindrance:

- **Positive transfer** tends to occur when the skills have a similar shape or form, such as the serving action of an overarm volleyball serve and a tennis serve.
- **Negative transfer** tends to occur when the skills appear to be similar at first glance but in fact are not identical, for example the difference in throwing action between a cricket return from the boundary (round arm) and a javelin throw (through the shoulder).

Other types of transfer include:
- **proactive transfer**, when a skill you already know is taken forward to affect a skill you are learning
- **retroactive transfer**, when a skill you have just been learning is taken back to affect one you already know.
- **bilateral transfer**, when a skill is moved across the body from limb to limb (e.g. when a basketball player who can do a lay up with the right hand learns to do it with the left hand)
- **zero transfer**, when two skills are so different that there is no chance of any correlation (e.g. rock climbing and swimming)

To ensure positive transfer, training sessions should be made as realistic as possible — for example, in hockey, rather than using cones you should use real players as defenders. You should work from the basics of the skill to the complexities, for example starting with the control of a netball before going on to making a pass, and giving praise when the player gets it right. Feedback could advise the players when transfer can be used and training could be centred on groups of skills requiring similar abilities, such as passing and catching and throwing drills that require coordination.

6 Schema theory

Schema theory is similar to the theory of transfer. It suggests that the same skills can be used in different sports because the performer has developed a general set of concepts that allows skills to be adapted to suit the situation. A schema is therefore a rule based on experience.

A motor programme that has been developed for a well-learned skill such as a netball pass could be adapted using feedback, so that the pass could then be used in basketball. Further experience could allow the pass to be used in rugby so that, rather than a concrete, well-defined skill, the performer has a set of concepts available to suit a variety of situations.

In order to operate the concepts of a schema, the performer must go through four processes:

(1) recognise the initial conditions, i.e. take in information from the environment about where he or she is (e.g. behind the line in basketball about to take a free throw)
(2) understand the response specifications, or 'what to do' (e.g. he or she is required to shoot the basketball at the ring)
(3) acknowledge the sensory consequences or the feel of the skill; in other words, take in information from the senses needed to complete the task (e.g. feeling the basketball in his or her hand as the shot is taken)
(4) judge the response outcome or result (e.g. was the shot successful?)

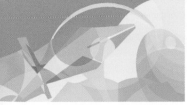
Parts 1 and 2 are derived from the memory or the motor programme and are therefore called the **recall schema**. They initiate the movement.

Parts 3 and 4 use feedback to adapt the motor programme and are therefore called the **recognition schema**. They control the movement.

A summary of schema theory is given in Figure 47. It shows how the motor programme is adapted using feedback to produce a more general concept.

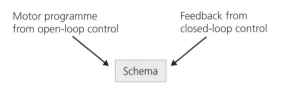

Figure 47

To develop a schema, coaches should vary practice to generate experience. They could point out when a schema can be used and then apply positive reinforcement when it is used successfully. Gradual progress from the early parts of the skill to the more complex parts should be made, and feedback should be used continuously to provide information on how to adapt the skill.

7 *Learning curves*

A learning curve is a graphic illustration that shows how a performer's rate of learning a closed skill can vary over a period of time. A typical learning curve looks like the one in Figure 48 and can be divided into four stages:

- At **stage A**, the rate of learning is slow and performance level is poor. This is because the performer is new to the task and is in the cognitive stage of learning, working out the required sub-routines and possibly using trial and error.
- At **stage B**, there is a rapid acceleration in the rate of learning because the performer has begun to master the task and gain some success, providing reinforcement and motivation.
- At **stage C**, there is no improvement in the rate of learning, and the performance has reached a 'plateau'. The **plateau effect** could be due to the fact that the performer has reached the limit of his or her ability, or is beginning to suffer from fatigue and lose some of the initial motivation. Alternatively, coaching may not be up to standard, resulting in poor technique, or the performer may have set his or her targets too low.
- At **stage D**, there is a drop in the rate of improvement and the performance may actually start to get worse, a concept called **drive reduction**. Drive reduction occurs because the performer has gained success at the task and the initial drive to succeed has been lost; the challenge of mastering the task has been overcome, and a new challenge or extension to the task is needed to maintain motivation.

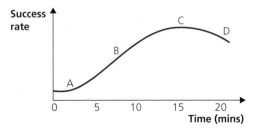

Figure 48

To overcome the reductions in performance at stages C and D, the coach should point out the plateau concept to the performer, so that the slowdown in improvement is understood, and use reinforcement, such as rewards and praise, to maintain motivation. The performer may be given a break to offset fatigue. A new coach could take over the training, and the player could reset his or her goals for the task.

Examiner's tip

Exam questions often refer to the three phases of learning and you must make sure that you can describe the key characteristics of each stage and give examples. Make sure that you differentiate between the cognitive *phase* of learning and the cognitive *theory* of learning — under exam pressure it is easy to misinterpret a question and write about the wrong topic. Know the difference between positive and negative reinforcement, namely that positive reinforcement involves a pleasant stimulus such as praise for a correct response, and negative reinforcement means taking away that praise for an incorrect response. Learn Thorndike's laws so you are able to show how to make the S–R bond stronger, and make sure you know the difference between positive and negative transfer and can give an appropriate example. The four parts of schema theory should be learned well so that you can recall them 'parrot fashion', should you be asked to do so.

There are many technical terms associated with the theories of learning, so make a checklist of them all as you revise to make sure you know them. A description of each term is usually worth a mark in the exam.

Please note that learning curves are not included in the OCR specification.

6 Teaching, practice and guidance

By the end of this topic, you should:
- understand the factors a coach must consider before attempting to teach a skill
- know the different styles of teaching and practising and when it is best to use these styles
- be able to link theory to practice by giving examples of each of the teaching and practice methods

1 Before teaching or practising

Before a coach attempts to undertake any practice session, there are some important considerations to be taken into account. These can be divided into two categories: concerns about the task and concerns about the performer.

1.1 Concerns about the task

The coach should consider the type of skill and make some attempt to classify it. Questions that should be asked include:
- Is it an open or closed skill?
- Does the skill require varied practice or fixed practice?
- Is the skill externally or internally paced, i.e. should the coach put the performers under pressure or leave them to do it in their own time?
- Is the skill discrete, requiring fast, whole practice, or is it continuous and the performers should be given a rest?
- Can the skill be broken down into parts?
- Is it a serial skill, which may require practising each part of the task?
- Is there any danger?
- How much time is available to complete the task?
- What facilities and equipment are available?
- How complex is the task?

1.2 Concerns about the performer

The abilities of participants should also be considered when deciding appropriate activities. For example:
- those with good coordination can complete complex passing drills
- those who are well motivated and fit can practise without a rest

Consideration should be made for:
- the age of the group
- the mix of males/females
- the fitness levels
- the motivation of the players

The experience of the performers should also be considered: experts should be able to repeat their drills and fine-tune their performance, while beginners should undertake a variety of practices.

Finally, the size of the group should be considered — a large group may have to be told to do the same thing because there is no time to concentrate on individuals.

2 Teaching styles

Having considered all of the above factors, the coach can then choose to adopt one of the following three teaching styles:

- command style
- reciprocal style
- problem-solving style

2.1 Command style

The command style is used by a coach who makes all the decisions and adopts an **authoritarian** approach. It is best used:

- when there is danger involved (e.g. telling a class of children not to dive into the shallow end of the swimming pool)
- for large groups, as it retains tight control
- when there is only one way of doing a task

It is an efficient method of teaching and therefore useful when the coach has little time or needs to meet deadlines.

A problem with the command style is that it does not cater for different abilities: a performer who is unable to do the set task may lose motivation and feel inferior, while someone who can extend the task beyond the range of movement being asked of them could also feel demotivated. No interaction between members of the group is allowed in this style.

2.2 Reciprocal style

The reciprocal style of teaching is used when there is a mix of abilities within the group and the teacher decides to set the tasks for the lesson and hand over part of the teaching to the more able performers. For example, a swimming coach who is unable to enter the water may ask expert swimmers to demonstrate starts and turns for less able members of the group.

The reciprocal style has several advantages:

- It promotes communication and interaction within the group.
- It may generate new ideas for the coach.
- It may aid the personal development of the more able performers.
- It gives immediate feedback to the group.

However, the reciprocal approach is time consuming, and there is a danger that the more able performers may lack coaching skills and present incorrect information to the others.

2.3 Problem-solving style

This is also known as the 'discovery style' and is used when the teacher sets a task for performers to complete in their own way. For example, a gym coach may ask the group to work out ways of travelling across a mat.

This teaching style:

- promotes group interaction
- allows performers to work at their own level, so that they can either extend their skills to more complex moves or complete the task in a simple way
- allows all levels of performer to succeed and gain motivation and satisfaction

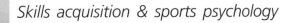

However, the problem-solving style is time consuming and, without teacher control, incorrect results may be achieved and dangerous techniques could be developed.

3 *Types of practice*

When deciding which type of practice to use, information about the task and the performers should be taken into consideration. The coach may opt for one of the following methods:
- whole practice
- part pratice
- fixed practice
- varied practice
- massed practice
- distributed practice
- mental practice

3.1 Whole practice

Whole practice means that the skill is performed in its entirety to promote fluency and to establish the links between each part of the task. It is used when the skill is ballistic or fast and highly organised, and cannot be broken down into its parts, for example a golf swing.

This method:
- promotes an understanding of the links between each sub-routine (e.g. the timing of the strike after the toss of the ball during a tennis serve)
- enables the performer to develop a feel for the whole task
- provides a more realistic method of practice
- achieves consistency in the execution of the skill, so that motor programmes are developed

The whole practice method may be good for simple skills that can easily be recalled or for advanced performers who are making skills habitual.

3.2 Part practice

The **whole–part–whole** method of practice can be used to highlight a weakness in performance, or when a complex task, or a task that is hard to break down, is being performed by a beginner. The task is performed in its entirety and the areas of weakness are then identified and practised separately. Once these components are improved, they are integrated back into the whole task.

The part method involves the skill being broken down into its sub-routines and practised separately before being put back together. There are two part methods:
- The **pure part method** is used to teach the skill one part at a time, and the parts are then put together at the end of the session. It is used when the skill is easily broken down, complex or dangerous, such as when the arm action, leg action and body positioning of a swimming stroke are taught separately during swimming drills.
- The **progressive part method** is used when the parts of the skill are added together in sequence as they are being taught. Sometimes called **chaining**, this method is used for serial skills, when the links between each part need to be established, or when there is danger. An example is each move in a trampolining routine being practised and linked to the move that precedes it.

The part methods of practice can:

- provide motivation
- build confidence
- reduce danger
- give an initial understanding of the task
- highlight weaknesses in technique and allow specific focus on these elements
- reduce demands on the performer and offset fatigue

The problems with the part methods are that they are time-consuming and, in the case of pure part practice, links between the sub-routines may be ignored. Sometimes students also may fail to get a feel for the whole task. The coach must try to avoid negative transfer between each part of the task.

3.3 Fixed practice

Fixed practice uses repetition of the same activity to promote **overlearning**. This ensures that more advanced performers maintain consistency in their performance and that their responses are habitual.

Fixed practice is appropriate:

- for closed skills
- when there is an element of danger
- when the skill is simple

An example is an experienced player practising a number of tennis serves from the same place on the court. The problem of boredom and fatigue can occur if this type of practice is used too much.

3.4 Varied practice

Varied practice is appropriate for beginners or when a coach needs to motivate performers. It helps performers to develop a **schema** and builds the sub-routines of the skill. It is appropriate for open skills or complex tasks when one element of the performance can be integrated with other aspects. An example is a group of beginners practising different passing and catching drills in a team sport.

Varied practice is time consuming, and the coach should avoid the possibility of negative transfer occurring.

3.5 Massed practice

Massed practice is used by a coach who wishes to promote a high degree of fitness in the players and make sure that the skill becomes 'grooved' and habitual. It is suitable for:

- expert performers who wish to maintain a degree of **autonomy** in their performance
- experts honing discrete skills, as the performer has no rest intervals in between practice sessions

An example is a professional footballer practising advanced passing drills without a break. However, the coach should try to avoid fatigue.

3.6 Distributed practice

Distributed practice allows the coach to grant a rest interval between practice sessions. It is appropriate for beginners as it lets the performer recuperate, and the rest interval can be used to offer feedback or to allow mental rehearsal of the set task. This places less stress and pressure on the performer.

This method provides motivation and can reduce danger because complex or risky elements of the task can be explained. An example is a footballer learning a basic passing drill, having a break and then going on to perform the drill against opposition.

3.7 Mental practice

Also called mental rehearsal, this increasingly popular technique involves a performer going over the routine in his or her mind, without moving. It has the effect of improving performance more than if just physical practice is undertaken.

Mental practice:
- improves confidence
- helps to control arousal
- develops the ability to think
- eliminates errors
- improves reaction time
- activates muscle receptors, giving sound preparation for the task ahead

Coaches can help beginners by leading them through the basic coaching points verbally and asking them to focus on these points during short periods of concentration. Performers can then go on to rehearse the next phases of the skill for increasingly longer periods of time. The first part of the skill should be learned thoroughly before progress is made.

For expert performers, mental rehearsal has the benefit of highlighting tactics or strategies and focusing on the opposition's weaknesses. Once the technique has been incorporated into the training programme, advanced performers should be able to control mental rehearsal themselves. It helps to maintain a high level of autonomous performance.

Ideally, mental rehearsal should be done in a relaxed environment, and the coach and player should concentrate only on success.

4 Guidance

Guidance methods are techniques used in conjunction with practice to help the performer with movement patterns.

4.1 Visual guidance

Visual guidance is when a coach uses an accurate demonstration to create a mental image of the task. It is especially useful for beginners, in that it can show aspects of technique or highlight weaknesses. A role model could be used to draw attention to the correct skills, but the coach should be careful to ensure that the performer is capable of actually doing the demonstration as shown or confidence could be affected.

4.2 Verbal guidance

Verbal guidance is best applied in conjunction with visual guidance, offering an explanation of the required movement to accompany the demonstration. It can be used for advanced performers to give tactical instruction and feedback on weaknesses. Any comments made by the coach should be brief and relevant so that the players can understand them and so that there is not too much information to take in at once.

4.3 Manual and mechanical guidance

More physical types of guidance are manual guidance and mechanical guidance:

- Manual guidance typically involves a coach using his or her hands to manipulate the athlete to perform the correct movements (e.g. giving support to a gymnast trying to perform a vault or a hand stand).
- Mechanical guidance is a device used to support the athlete, such as a swimming armband or a harness on the trampoline.

Manual or mechanical guidance should be used early in skill development, since they provide early confidence, reduce danger and allow an early feel for the task to develop. However, these forms of guidance should be withdrawn as progress is made, since the performer may become dependent on them and begin to feel that they are unable to do the task without the help, actually causing a loss in motivation. If used too much, these physical types of guidance may begin to interfere with the internal feel of the whole unaided movement.

Examiner's tip

Exam questions often ask you to name the elements you should consider before practising a skill. Make sure that you differentiate between considerations associated with the task and those associated with the performer. For example, the level of motivation concerns the performer, not the task. Try not to confuse styles of teaching (command, reciprocal and problem-solving) with the types of practice, and make sure that you can give examples from practical activities for every type of practice or teaching style.

Exam candidates often fail to gain the maximum marks because they repeat the same point. If you stated that the command style of teaching eliminates danger and that the problem-solving style may result in dangerous situations, you would only get 1 mark. However, if you said that the command style has the advantage of eliminating danger whereas the problem-solving style has the disadvantage of being time-consuming, you would get 2 marks. Make sure you know the reasons why mental rehearsal improves performance and how experts and beginners use mental rehearsal in different ways. This is often asked as a more testing question in the latter part of the exam.

Please note that teaching styles do not form part of the OCR specification.

TOPIC 7 Motivation and arousal

By the end of this topic, you should:
- understand the terminology associated with the concepts of motivation and arousal in sport
- know the theories that relate arousal to performance
- be able to recognise methods that a coach would use to motivate performers

1 Motivation

Motivation is an inner drive. It is defined as the external stimuli and internal mechanisms that arouse and direct behaviour. There are two types of motivation:
- **Extrinsic motivation** comes from an outside source, such as praise from a coach or the incentive of winning a badge or trophy.
- **Intrinsic motivation** is an inner drive to achieve success and derives from a pride and satisfaction in completing a task or a determination to achieve personal goals.

Extrinsic motivation lays the foundation for future effort and can be used to attract newcomers to an activity. For example, the 'Duckling' awards are a means of promoting swimming activity among toddlers. However, if awards were given out all the time they would lose their motivational effect, since the performer would become familiar with them. Rewards need to be made increasingly difficult in order to maintain motivation. Intrinsic motivation, such as the setting of personal goals, should be used as the performer gains experience, so that motivation levels remain constant.

A coach could motivate a player by:
- offering praise, positive feedback or positive reinforcement
- ensuring that success is achieved early and that tasks are then gradually made more difficult
- breaking the skill down into parts so that success is attained in each part, and making the performer feel responsible for each success
- setting realistic targets
- pointing out both role models and the health benefits of the activity

2 Arousal

Arousal is the degree to which we are activated and ready to perform the task ahead. A large audience, the challenge of a new activity or the incentive of a major reward such as a trophy or medal could cause an increase in the level of arousal in sport. There are three theories that link the level of arousal to the level of performance:
- drive theory
- drive reduction theory
- inverted-U theory

2.1 Drive theory

Drive theory maintains that as our level of arousal increases, so our performance improves, in a **linear** or constant fashion. It is explained by the formula: $P = D \times H$.

This means that performance is equal to drive multiplied by habit. The theory suggests that:

- we are initially motivated by the challenge of meeting the task or by the 'big game'
- the increased effort we put in brings us more success and a stronger drive to continue performing
- success provides reinforcement, and we carry on repeating the successful responses so that the performance becomes habitual

Drive theory is illustrated in Figure 49.

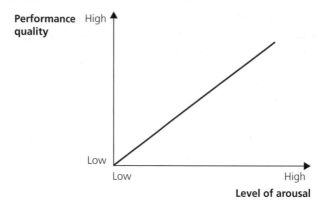

Figure 49

However, at high levels of arousal the ability to take in information from the environment is reduced and we may only focus on the **dominant response** or most intense stimulus. Expert performers may be able to continue playing well at high arousal because they can focus on the correct dominant response, but a novice could focus on an incorrect response and performance could suffer.

2.2 Drive reduction theory

Drive reduction theory suggests that motivation is high at the start of the learning process, when we are challenged by the need to master the task; however, once we have succeeded, our initial drive is lost — the need has been satisfied. A new challenge or an extension to the skill is required to provide further motivation.

2.3 Inverted-U theory

Inverted-U theory is more realistic and states that increased arousal will improve performance to a point, or **optimum peak**, that occurs at some level of moderate arousal. Further increases in arousal cause performance to deteriorate, so that both under- and over-arousal can result in a performance that is below par. Figure 50 illustrates the inverted-U theory.

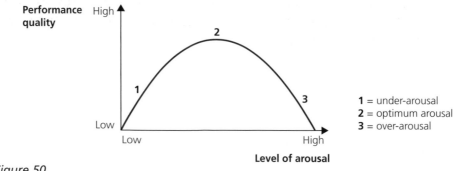

Figure 50

The optimum arousal level needed to produce the best performance can vary, and is dependent on the task and the performer:

- A gross skill needs less control than a fine skill and so requires a higher level of arousal.
- A complex task requires the performer to process a large amount of information; this is done more easily at lower levels of arousal. Conversely, a simple task is best performed at high arousal.
- Novices find it difficult to operate at high levels of arousal, as they are not able to cope with increased pressure.
- Experts still perform well at high levels of arousal, as they have the experience to select the right cues under pressure.

The influence of the task and the performer could make the inverted-U graph look different. A modified version is shown in Figure 51.

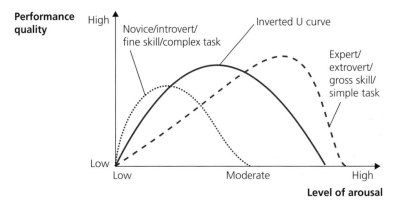

Figure 51

Examiner's tip

Questions on motivation usually focus either on an explanation of the difference between extrinsic and intrinsic motivation, or on the methods you could use to motivate a sports performer. Make sure that you have a sound knowledge of these areas and that you can use examples from sport to illustrate them.

If you are required to answer questions on drive theory or the inverted-U theory, your first step should be to draw a diagram showing the relationship between arousal and performance. If you answer questions on the inverted-U theory, make sure that you point out that under- and over-arousal can produce a below-par performance and that the optimum performance occurs at a moderate level. Make sure you can describe how both the task and the performer can modify the shape of the inverted U. You will usually gain a mark for the drive theory formula $(P = D \times H)$. Don't forget to include the fact that, according to this theory, at high arousal we focus on the dominant response and performance could be hindered.

By the end of this topic, you should:
- be able to explain the theories relating personality, attitudes and aggression to sport
- be aware of the nature and nurture approaches in explaining the development of individual characteristics in sport
- be able to suggest practical applications of the concepts of personality, attitudes and aggression in sport

1 *Personality*

Personality can be defined as a person's unique characteristics. These characteristics make individuals behave differently in sporting situations. There are three theories that try to explain how personality characteristics develop:
- trait theory
- social learning theory
- interactionist theory

1.1 Theories of personality

1.1a Trait theory

Trait theory suggests that we are born with personality characteristics or traits that are stable and enduring, so that we tend to behave in the same way in most situations. According to trait theory, it is therefore possible to predict how a performer will behave, and a profile of an individual can be developed to help coaches make predictions.

Eysenck developed a diagram (Figure 52) that showed extrovert (loud), introvert (reserved), neurotic (extreme) and stable (consistent) characteristics.

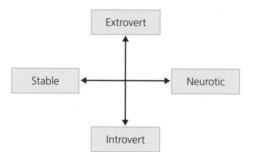

Figure 52

According to the diagram, an individual can, for example, be classed as a 'stable extrovert', i.e. consistently behaving in a loud manner. Catell developed a similar personality inventory to predict behaviour; it showed 16 source characteristics and the secondary characteristics of extroversion, independence, toughness and anxiety.

The problem with such personality profiles is that they are poor at predicting behaviour:
- The results of questionnaires can be unreliable and inconsistent, often producing varying results for the same individual using the same test at different times. Individuals can sometimes misunderstand the questions.

- Players often behave differently outside the game to how they behave within the sports arena, and even at different times in the game their behaviour can change. For example, a player may have an unpredictable reaction to a foul.

1.1b Social learning theory

Social learning theory suggests that personality traits are developed from our experiences and association with others — we can learn our behaviour from role models or from significant others such our parents and friends. We perceive our associates' behaviour as normal and adopt it as our own, a concept known as the **socialisation process**.

Behaviour is more likely to be learned if it is reinforced, powerful and consistent, such as the flamboyant goal celebrations of professional footballers copied by young players. Social learning theory suggests that our behaviour changes with the situation and that we do not behave in the same way all the time.

1.1c Interactionist theory

Interactionist theory combines trait and social learning approaches to personality by stating that we are born with traits that are then adapted to the situation. Our behaviour therefore changes with the situation and can be explained by the formula $B = f(P \times E)$, where behaviour is a function of personality multiplied by environment. A boxer who is calm outside the ring would be aggressive and forceful when in competition.

1.2 Personality measures

Psychologists have tried to measure personality in three ways:

- A **questionnaire** has the advantage of dealing with lots of information quickly and efficiently. A question may, however, be misunderstood, and performers could give answers they think they ought to give rather than telling the truth.
- Sporting **behaviour can be observed** to assess personality; a true picture can be gained, especially if the performer is unaware of the observation. However, the results of such observations are open to interpretation by the observer and are therefore subjective.
- Personality can be measured by some form of **physiological response** to exercise, such as heart rate. This is an objective measure, so the results can be used to make comparisons during performance. However, performers might not take kindly to the restrictions imposed by the measuring equipment in a real game, and knowledge that they are being measured can cause stress and distort results.

1.3 Profile of mood states (POMS)

One piece of research into sports personality attempted to link athletes' mood to their performance. Successful and less successful athletes were given a questionnaire about how they felt when taking part in major sporting events. The results are shown on the graph below, which indicates that less successful athletes show little variation in feelings as they compete, with moderate scores in each mood state. Successful athletes show similar scores to less successful athletes except for the quality of vigour, for which they score highly. This gives an 'iceberg' shape to the profile on the graph (see Figure 53).

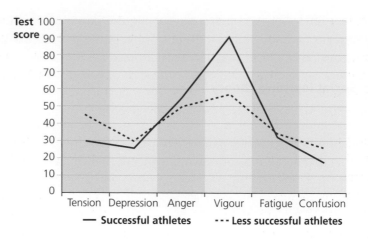

Figure 53

1.4 Achievement motivation

Achievement motivation is a concept of personality that tells us how competitive we are. The psychologist Atkinson suggested that there are two types of personality related to sport:

- The first type comprises performers who enjoy competition, take responsibility for their actions, welcome feedback to help them improve and do not mind taking risks. Such people are competitive and put their success down to their own efforts. They are motivated by the **need to achieve**, or 'Nach'. A performer motivated by the need to achieve tries harder after failure, e.g. a swimmer who just fails to reach his or her personal best time in a race will try harder in training to achieve the time in the next race.

- The second type comprises those who take easy options, do not take responsibility for their actions and prefer not to use feedback — they are motivated by the **need to avoid failure**, or 'Naf'. A performer motivated by the need to avoid failure tends to give up after failure, e.g. a squash player who has lost a few games may abandon his or her attempt to move up the club ladder.

The concepts of Nach and Naf are summarised in Figure 54, which shows that the ideal performer in sport should have a high Nach and low Naf.

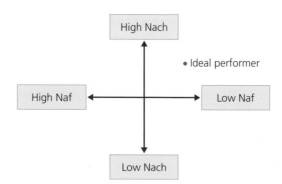

Figure 54

The development of the competitive instinct, or the need to achieve, is said to occur in three stages:

- The **autonomous competence stage** is when a young performer is concerned with simply mastering the task. For example, can a simple catch or throw be completed successfully?

- In the **social comparison stage**, occurring from the age of approximately 6 years, the youngster not only performs the skill but also tries to compare his or her efforts with others, so that the length of a throw compared with that of a friend is important.
- In the **integrated or more adult stage**, all forms of internal and external standards are used to gauge performance, so that a netball player would judge her game on her own feel for the skill and on feedback from the coach.

These three stages suggest that a Nach approach to sport is based on initial competitive traits that are developed by access to coaching and the opportunity to play and gain experience. Coaches should try to ensure that their athletes continue to have the **motivation to succeed** by allowing initial success and giving rewards and praise to beginners. They could maintain confidence as the athletes develop by pointing out early failure as a means to improvement, or by redefining failure not as a measure of winning and losing but as a measure of personal improvement. Successful role models could be noted, and anxiety levels could be lowered through the use of relaxation techniques. The performers should feel that there is enough incentive value in completing the task. Tasks that are difficult to achieve but produce a sense of satisfaction when completed offer real motivation. Easy tasks that are below the performers' capability present little incentive.

2 Attitudes

Attitudes are mental states of expectation directed towards something. Our attitudes comprise three parts:
- the **cognitive part** includes beliefs, such as those about the benefits of exercise
- the **affective part** concerns feelings and interpretation of beliefs — for example, we might enjoy exercise
- the **behavioural part** is about actions taken — for example, we may take part in sport and train regularly

However, we may not always behave according to our beliefs. We might believe that weight training makes us stronger, but if strength were not necessary for our chosen sport, we would not do any strength training. The affective part of the attitude determines our judgement.

2.1 Formation of attitudes

Attitudes can develop from:
- **past experiences** (from which an attitude is *learned*)
- **association with significant others** (people we hold in high esteem, such as friends, role models or coaches)
- **media sources**, such as newspapers

Attitudes are often based on our beliefs and can be positive or negative:
- **Positive attitudes** can be formed by positive past experiences, such as enjoyable games in which we played well and which gave us confidence. We may enjoy the challenge of sport and see it as stress release. If the people we associate with regularly are keen on sport, we also tend to be more positive about sport.
- **Negative attitudes** can develop if we have had a bad experience, such as an injury, if we feel anxiety or stress when taking part in sport, if the people we associate with are non-sporty or if we feel we lack ability.

2.2 Changing attitudes

Coaches would like the attitudes of their players to be positive, and it is sometimes necessary to change negative attitudes. The process of **cognitive dissonance** can do this by challenging a player's beliefs. It might be possible to persuade a rugby player to do some aerobics, if you suggest that aerobics is a measure of true stamina and that an hour-long session can be more demanding than the player anticipates.

Persuasion is more effective if it is delivered by an expert — if a physiotherapist or a coach initiated the above conversation about aerobics, it might have more impact than if it had been suggested by someone who does not play sport. A coach could change negative attitudes by:

- pointing out the benefits of exercise
- allowing the players to gain initial success as beginners
- making training sessions enjoyable
- encouraging players with rewards and praise

2.3 Prejudice

A prejudice is a more extreme attitude created by media hype or by our desire to fit in with a group — a form of social pressure. We may give undue weight to a bad experience and develop a negative attitude as a result of it. Examples of prejudice in sport include negative thoughts towards officials, older players, players of a different race or gender, or a positive feeling for our own team. The crowd at an important football game may become incensed when the referee makes a poor decision and gives a penalty to the opposition that decides the game. If members of the crowd shout abuse at the referee, it is likely that we will join in with the abuse in order to fit in with the other supporters' behaviour.

To prevent prejudice in sport, cognitive dissonance or persuasion may be used, and the coach could reinforce players' fair behaviour with rewards. Role models from alternative racial groups or from the opposite gender may be introduced, and during training the coach might mix groups of different gender or ethnic background in order to widen players' experience.

2.4 Aggression in sport

The level of individual aggression displayed in sport can vary. One problem of looking at aggression is the confusion over a clear definition. Some sports commentators often confuse aggression with **assertion**:

- Aggression is the intent to harm, often outside the rules of the game. It is an out-of-control reaction to, say, a bad foul in football.
- Assertion is more controlled behaviour that is within the rules and lacks intent to injure, such as a hard but fair rugby tackle.

Even within the confines of these definitions, it is difficult to classify some sports in terms of aggression. In boxing, for example, it is within the rules to hit an opponent to cause harm. A summary of the definitions of aggression and assertion is given in Figure 55, showing a grey area where some aspects may overlap.

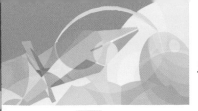
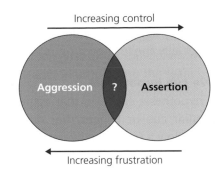

Figure 55

There are four theories that attempt to explain how aggression is caused in sport:
- instinct theory
- the frustration–aggression (F–A) hypothesis
- social learning theory
- the aggressive cue hypothesis

2.4a Instinct theory

Instinct theory claims that we all have an aggressive trait as part of our nature, developed from our ancestors as a result of a survival instinct. This may surface in sport if circumstances, such as being fouled, cause us to react. Some performers do not need much provocation to react aggressively, while others do not react so easily.

2.4b The frustration–aggression (F–A) hypothesis

The frustration–aggression (F–A) hypothesis (see Figure 56) states that aggression is an inevitable consequence of frustrating circumstances when our goals or intentions are blocked. If the aggression is released and the player is allowed to let off steam, a tense situation could be resolved quickly. For example, a football player who is fouled while bearing down on the goal might punch the player who fouled him and then calm down.

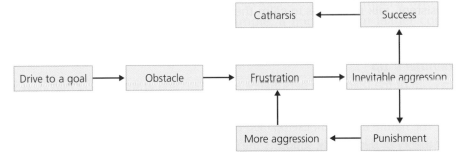

Figure 56

However, if the aggressive instinct is not released, for example if the referee prevents retaliation for the foul, it may be harboured and an even more aggressive act could occur later. The release of the aggressive instinct is known as **catharsis**, derived from a Greek term meaning 'cleansing the emotions'.

2.4c Social learning theory

Social learning theory claims that our aggressive responses are not just instinctive, but can be learned from our experiences and from witnessing the behaviour of significant others. Imagine a basketball player who sees her captain foul an opponent she is marking closely, as a result of which the opposing player is put off her game. The

A leader may use other styles:

- The **social support style** is used in a one-on-one situation by a coach to discuss a player's performance; it is popular because it offers feedback.
- The **rewarding style** might be used with beginners to offer incentives such as praise, and is preferred by players because of the obvious motivational features.
- A **training and instruction style** is what many coaches do best — performance is improved in a structured manner with skills and drills, and players are aware of the benefits of this style.
- A **laissez faire style** of leadership is a relaxed approach, where the leader allows the group to act independently, and is only appropriate for experienced players who know what they are doing.

1.2 Choice of style

The style chosen by the leader depends on three main factors:

- The situation often predetermines the best style to use, so that in a dangerous activity the leader would be autocratic. If the task involved interactive team sports, a training and instruction style might be appropriate.
- Leaders may choose the style that they are most used to and comfortable with, according to their personality and characteristics. For example, an extrovert with good communication skills would probably use a training and instruction style.
- Groups want to be led in a certain style. Beginners need to be instructed, while experts may wish to discuss issues. A large group must be instructed in an autocratic manner since there is insufficient time to cater for all the group members; conversely, coaching an individual may allow time for some social support.

Chelladurai stated that a satisfactory and enjoyable performance is achieved if there is harmony between the situation, the leader's chosen style and the group requirements. Figure 58 shows that the more the leader's actual behaviour meets the expectations of the group and the demands of the situation, the better the performance.

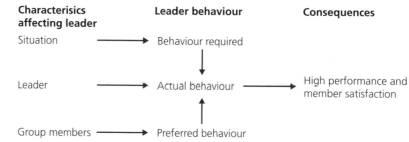

Figure 58

The nature/nurture debate can also occur in leadership. Leaders may be born with innate leadership qualities, such as communication skills. On the other hand, a leader might learn to be a sports captain through experience and by copying role models. Interactionist theory would argue that good leaders have the necessary traits and use them in the required situation. A good leader could therefore adapt to the situation, motivating the team members when they are losing and listening to them when they need advice.

2 *Team dynamics*

A group can be defined as a collection of people who mutually interact in order to achieve a common goal. In sport, a team is a classic example of a group, as the players have to interact with each other to gain success. Two sprint athletes who train at the same time but for different events do not qualify as a group, but when they are put together in a relay team their interaction at the baton change becomes important. A sports group is said to form in four stages:

- Stage 1 is the **forming stage**. The group members meet and begin to establish identities and roles, getting to know each other.
- Stage 2 is the **storming stage**. Rivalries and conflicts may develop, e.g. the realisation that two players want to play in the same position.
- Stage 3 is the '**norming**' stage. Earlier conflicts are resolved, e.g. the two players may now agree to change their positions to help the team.
- Stage 4 is a **performing stage**. The team carries out the task and attempts to achieve success.

The type of sport can affect **cohesion** (the desire to reach a common goal):

- **Individual sports**, such as athletics, do not require much cohesion (unless the athlete is part of a relay race).
- **Co-active sports**, which involve a pair (e.g. a doubles team in badminton), require more cohesion.
- **Interactive sports**, such as football, need the highest level of cohesion.

The achievements of a team in sport are affected by a number of processes that can be summed up by the formula: $AP = PP - FP$, where actual productivity is equal to potential productivity minus faulty processes.

This formula means that what the group actually achieves is equal to the best performance it could give minus the influences on the team that cause things to go wrong. The elements that can go wrong are important for the sports psychologist to understand and include problems with **coordination**, **cohesion** and **motivation**.

2.1 Coordination and cohesion problems within a team

Coordination problems occur when the team members or the coach get it wrong. This may be because the tactics were incorrect or because the players misunderstood the coach's instructions. For example, a basketball team may have lost a game because it used a one-on-one defence when a zonal system would have been more appropriate.

A more serious problem occurs when the team lacks cohesion. Two types of cohesion have been identified:

- **Task cohesion** concerns the result and achievement of the group.
- **Social cohesion** concerns how the personalities within the team get on with each other.

Sometimes, players can put aside personality clashes for the sake of achieving an important result, so in a sense task cohesion can override social cohesion. Both types of cohesion are said to contain two elements:

- The **attraction element** is what drew you to the group in the first place — in sport, this is likely to mean an enjoyment of working as a unit to meet challenges.
- The **integration element** is what then happens when you are in the group, i.e. how you get on with other members of the team.

A summary of the types of cohesion is illustrated in Figure 59.

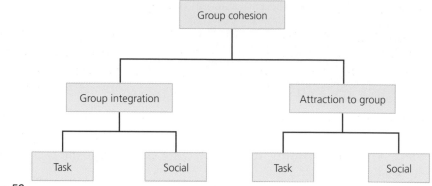

Figure 59

Within any team there are a number of factors that affect the level of cohesion shown by the players:

- Integration can be affected by **personality**. If all the players were extroverts, it would be difficult for them to get on because they might all want the limelight.
- Players on **unequal pay** might not get on. A new player brought into a professional team could upset existing players if he or she is on a higher level of pay.
- Team members who have regular **social opportunities** may become more prepared to work for each other in a game.
- If the players share the **same goals** and have **similar values**, it is more likely that they will strive to succeed. A team that has a chance of winning the league will have the unified goal of success.
- Good **communication skills** can help to eliminate coordination problems, for example if players identify and discuss an opponent they will be marking.
- The motivational qualities of the **group leader** are important in promoting unity. The coach or captain should identify roles and tactics clearly before the game.
- **External threats** can often bind a team together. A team being investigated by the sport's governing body for rule infringements may collectively decide to prove itself on the field of play.

There are several ways of tackling coordination and cohesion problems:

- A coach could use knowledge of the factors influencing cohesion to promote team building.
- Common team goals could be set, such as qualifying for the end-of-season play-offs.
- In training, the coach could use interactive drills that encourage the players both to communicate and to work together.
- A coach could ensure that tactics are outlined clearly.
- Team social events could be arranged.
- Wearing team colours to matches could help develop a group identity.

2.1a Cohesion and success

Trends would show that successful teams are usually more cohesive; or is it that cohesive teams are more successful? There is no doubt that social cohesion promotes integration, but it is not enough on its own. Task cohesion is more important in making the players strive for success, and even individual differences within the team can be forgotten when there is a goal to aim for. Task cohesion can be enough to promote success without social cohesion, but the most successful teams show both task and social cohesion in their performances.

2.2 Motivational problems within a team

The psychologist Ringlemann carried out an observation of participants in a tug-of-war competition. He found that the more group members involved in pulling on the rope, the less the individual effort. A group of eight did not pull with the force of eight times one individual. He concluded that group performance reduced with group size.

One of the reasons for this reduced effort could be that within a team, individuals can hide and blame others for poor team performance. The tendency of individuals to reduce their efforts within a team is called **social loafing**. This phenomenon tends to occur when:

- team members think that their efforts are not being recognised and subsequently lose motivation, i.e. lack of **performance identification**
- players are offered little encouragement, i.e. poor leadership
- players have a fear of failure or are worried they are being watched closely by, for example, a chief scout and are not prepared to take risks in case they make a mistake
- players lack confidence or do not believe in their ability; they tend to leave the major tasks in the game to others.
- players get the impression that others in the team are not trying and therefore lose the motivation to try themselves

Social loafing is not desirable, so knowledge of its causes can help a coach to prevent players losing motivation in future games. The coach should highlight individual performances with statistics and could use praise and rewards to raise confidence. Allowing success in early training sessions can develop belief in ability, and any success achieved should be put down to the skill of the performer. In training, the specific roles of the players should be made clear, and the team members should be encouraged to help each other.

Examiner's tip

The concepts of group dynamics relate strongly to team performances in real game situations, so you can expect questions to ask for practical examples. Make sure that every point you make can be backed up with an example from sport. Even if you are not asked for a specific example, including one in your answer may help you to gain a mark that you otherwise might not have achieved. The example may explain a key point, in which case the examiner should credit it.

Questions on leadership tend to require explanations of the Chelladurai and Fielder models, so make sure you know them well. Often the question will give you a diagram to interpret, such as the one that depicts the Chelladurai model. Do not be deterred by a diagram — simply take each part in turn and account for it. This will provide a structure for your answer.

Questions on sports groups often ask for details of specific concepts, such as social loafing, the Ringlemann effect and cohesion.

By the end of this topic, you should:
- understand the pressures that can affect a sports performer, both before and after a performance
- know how coaches and players deal with those pressures
- understand the motivational strategies a player can use to help improve performance

1 *Motivation*

You might recall from Topic 7 that motivation can be extrinsic or intrinsic:
- **Extrinsic motivation** comes from an outside source, such as praise from a coach or the incentive of an available reward, and should be used in the early stages of learning to develop interest in the activity. However, overuse of extrinsic rewards can lead to a loss in motivation because the player may become too familiar with them.
- **Intrinsic motivation** concentrates on personal improvement and is used as a more permanent method of motivating an experienced player. Some more advanced methods of motivating players individually are discussed in this topic.

1.1 Goal setting

One of the more consistent findings of research studies into sports psychology is the link between goal setting and improved performance. Players who set themselves targets or have goals set by the coach generally produce better results. This is because the goals provide personal motivation and a sense of satisfaction when a target is achieved. If goals are set within a player's reach, confidence can be improved, and a more difficult target set to allow further improvement. Goal setting also plays an important role in lowering anxiety and reducing the stress of performing at a high level.

The goals set by coaches and players can be long term or short term:
- **Long-term goals** are concerned with the end result of a lengthy period of work and are sometimes called **outcome goals**. An example would be a swimmer aiming to qualify for regional team selection by meeting the required time before next year's major championship.
- **Short-term goals** are the stepping-stones to meeting long-term targets. Short-term goals can be **performance-related**, or judged against a past performance. For example, an attempt by a swimmer to beat a personal best time by the end of next month is a step along the way to eventually meeting the regional target time. Short-term goals can also be **process-related** or concerned with technique; for example, in order to achieve a personal best, the swimmer must work on improving the exit from the turn.

A summary of the types of goals that can be set by players and coaches is given in Figure 60.

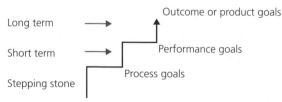

Figure 60

When setting such goals, it is important that coaches do not focus solely on winning. In a swimming race, for example, there can only be one winner and performers who

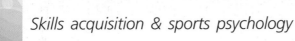
fail to meet the target may lose motivation and suffer stress. It is more important to set goals that can be achieved by everyone, such as those targets that focus on personal improvement and technique. You might not win the swimming race but you can still gain a personal best time and show improved technique.

Other factors that a coach should take into account when setting goals are summed up by the **SMARTER** principle. This set of guidelines is outlined as follows:

- **S = specific** — e.g. not just 'improve fitness', but run a specified distance 3 seconds faster
- **M = measured** — statistics or a stopwatch can tell you how you are doing
- **A = agreed** — sit down and discuss the goals with your coach
- **R = realistic** — the goals should offer a challenge but be achievable
- **T = timed** — give yourself a deadline to keep yourself focused; long or short term?
- **E = exciting** — you will work harder for something you are interested in
- **R = recorded** — write down your progress so you can evaluate how you are doing

Following these principles should result in improved performance and confidence.

2 Confidence

Confidence is defined as a belief in the ability to master a particular situation. It is related to the personality concepts discussed in Topic 8, especially in relation to the level of competitiveness or **achievement motivation** shown by the performer. If you are confident, you will try harder, take more risks and accept challenges more readily. Athletes who are low on confidence may suffer anxiety and be unprepared to accept competitive situations. In other words, confident performers have a high need to achieve, and players low in confidence may exhibit the need to avoid failure.

The level of confidence shown in any sporting situation is the product of a number of influences:

- **personality** — the traits you are born with are important, in that extroverts may be generally more confident and naturally more competitive
- **experience** — you will be more confident about succeeding in a situation you have mastered in the past; a belief in your ability may have been developed by success in training or in past performances
- **situation** — for example, you may feel a little more nervous before an important game in front of a large crowd, especially if it is the first time you have played in such conditions

Performers can display **trait confidence**, **state confidence** or (more likely) a combination of both. Trait confidence is a general disposition to be confident in most situations. State confidence is the belief in success in a particular situation, perhaps because you have succeeded in a similar situation in the past. A performer with trait confidence who also has confidence in a particular situation would be extremely self-assured of success. An experienced rugby player with trait confidence who is about to take part in the school house rugby competition would be confident of performing well.

2.1 Self-efficacy

The psychologist Albert Bandura refers to situation-specific self-confidence as 'self-efficacy', i.e. the strength of an individual's belief that he or she can successfully perform a given activity.

According to Bandura's research, the level of confidence shown by a sports performer is affected by four factors:

- **Performance accomplishments** refer to previous experiences and past successes. For example, if the bar in a high jump competition is at 1.25 m and you have jumped 1.6 m in training, you will be fairly confident of getting over the bar. Performance accomplishments can be promoted by setting easy targets and pointing out past successes.
- **Vicarious experiences** comprise what you have seen done by others that gives you confidence to undertake a task. An accurate demonstration from the coach is an example, as is watching someone from your peer group perform a difficult skill such as a gym vault. This gives you a clear vision of what to do. Vicarious experiences can also involve using a role model to show correct techniques.
- **Verbal persuasion** is the encouragement and praise you might receive from your coach, along the lines of: 'I know you can do this.'
- **Emotional arousal** refers to your level of anxiety and level of motivation before the event. Remaining calm under pressure will help performance. Emotional arousal can be controlled by using relaxation techniques and mental rehearsal or visualisation.

Coaches should use their knowledge of each of these aspects to ensure that performers face the situation with confidence.

3 *The relationship between arousal and performance*

Arousal is defined as the level of readiness to perform. It is an **energised** state that prepares the body for action, but too much or too little arousal can have a detrimental effect on performance. Increased arousal can be caused by:

- the approach of a major competition or big game
- others watching us perform (especially if those watching are knowledgeable about the sport or are known to us)
- increasingly frustrating circumstances, such as being fouled
- a fear of failure

The effect of arousal on performance is explained by the **inverted-U theory**. This states that increases in arousal improve performance up to a point, occurring at moderate arousal, but that further increases can have a detrimental effect (see Figure 61). The inverted-U theory can be adapted to suit different types of performer:

- Novices operate best at low arousal, as they are inexperienced in dealing with the pressures that an expert can cope with.
- An introvert needs little stimulation to provoke increases in arousal and therefore needs to keep arousal levels low, while an extrovert can tolerate an increased adrenaline rush.

The theory can also be adapted for different situations:

- A simple task requires little decision-making, and at high arousal fewer decisions are made; at low arousal, we may be more able to make the decisions necessary for complex skills.
- Gross skills can be performed at high arousal as they require less control than fine skills.

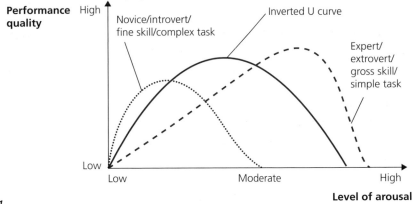

Figure 61

You should refer to the section on motivation and arousal to review the notes on the inverted-U theory, drive theory and drive reduction theory. Some of the theories discussed in this section are based on knowledge of the inverted-U theory and its concepts are therefore outlined in more detail.

3.1 Catastrophe theory

This adapted version of the inverted-U theory explains why a sporting performance can decline suddenly. Increases in arousal improve performance up to a point. However, after this point performance does not decline gradually. A further increase in arousal pushes the performer over the edge and performance falls dramatically. A small increase in arousal, caused perhaps by a worry about not playing well, by the threat of a difficult opponent or by playing in a major final in front of a big crowd, can have a **cumulative effect**. When added to existing arousal levels, this increase can cause a catastrophe even for experts.

If you scored from a penalty in the first half of a cup game but later in the game you were called on to take the final kick of the penalty shoot-out to decide who goes to the final, the increase in pressure may cause you to miss the penalty. To get over the catastrophe, the performer must return to a level of arousal that was present before the catastrophe occurred, a feat that is not always possible under extreme pressure.

Figure 62 illustrates catastrophe theory.

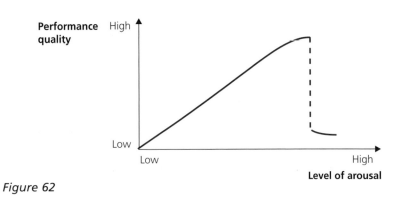

Figure 62

3.2 The zone of optimal functioning

The psychologist Hanin adapted the inverted-U theory. He suggested that increases in arousal can improve performance and that the optimal level of arousal does vary for individual players. However, rather than there being a **point** of optimal arousal, the best level of arousal for maximum confidence and control in sport is an area, or **zone**.

To achieve the zone can be the ultimate experience in sport, and performers can find their own zone using techniques such as mental rehearsal, relaxation, visualisation and positive self-talk. (These methods are discussed in more detail later in this section.) Once performers are in the zone, performance is said to improve because things seem to flow effortlessly. They reach a state of supreme confidence and remain calm under the utmost pressure. They feel that they are in total control of their actions and they are completely focused on the activity. The result is a smooth, effortless performance at the highest level. A diagram of the zone of optimal functioning is given in Figure 63.

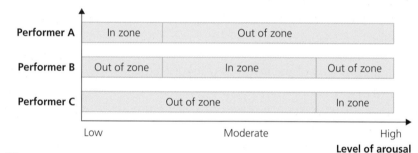

Figure 63

Performer A operates best at low arousal; a golfer, for example, needs control when about to make a putt. Performer B needs a moderate level of arousal. An example is a volleyball player making a block, a situation where whole body action is required but control is still needed. Performer C operates most effectively at high arousal; for example, a rugby player making a tackle needs real motivated effort.

3.3 The peak flow experience

The experience of being 'in the zone' can be enhanced if performers feel that the challenge of the task is appropriate to their level of skill. According to this theory:
- a player who has little skill and is presented with a difficult task would suffer anxiety (e.g. an inexperienced rock climber would be nervous if he/she were asked to ascend a difficult route)
- a player with little skill who is unable to complete a challenge would be apathetic towards the task
- a highly skilled player who is asked to do an easy task would become bored quickly (e.g. the young, experienced swimmer who trains 5 mornings a week would not relish the basic demands of a school swimming lesson for beginners)

Figure 64 illustrates these combinations.

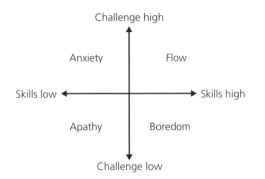

Figure 64

4 Attention

Devoting our attention to the activity in question is an important element of sports performance. Attention is defined as the ability to focus on the relevant environmental cues and is related to our level of arousal.

The **cue utilisation hypothesis** states:

- At **low arousal levels**, the attentional field of vision is wide and a performer is able to gather a large amount of information from the environment. However, this may cause confusion and deterioration in performance. The cue utilisation hypothesis offers another explanation of the inverted-U theory. Having too much information to process at one time is called **attention overload**. This causes the *perceptual field* to narrow and the performer to become distracted, perhaps scanning the playing field less often and attending to incorrect stimuli.
- At **high arousal levels**, the attentional field narrows and a performer is only able to focus on a limited amount of information, perhaps missing important cues. Only experienced performers are able to operate successfully at high arousal, and for others performance may suffer.
- At **moderate arousal**, we pick up and process relevant stimuli and disregard the irrelevant stimuli — further evidence to suggest that, in line with the inverted-U theory, a moderate level of arousal is best for peak performance. Coaches should try to control arousal levels with relaxation techniques to find the best operating level for their players.

Distraction-conflict theory suggests that the presence of a distraction, which could be from an external source such as the crowd or from an internal source such as worry about an injury, will cause internal conflict and an increase in arousal levels that could cause performance to deteriorate, especially if the performer is a beginner. The effect of distractions is made worse if the task being executed is complex or needs to be thought out carefully. Figure 65 summarises distraction-conflict theory.

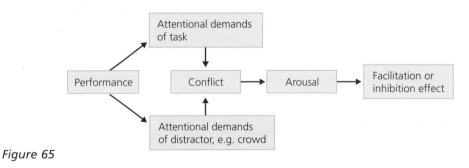

Figure 65

4.1 Attentional style

Niddefer suggested that a sports performer should choose the most appropriate style of picking up information from the environment. We have already examined how broad and narrow styles are adopted in sport, and Niddefer added the idea that these two styles could also be classed as internal or external.

Figure 66 indicates that four styles are possible:

	External	Internal
Broad	Position of players in game, e.g. a playmaker reading the game	Analyse and plan, e.g. coach tactics
Narrow	Focus on single cue, e.g. golf ball to hole	Mental rehearsal to control anxiety, e.g. focus on start

Figure 66

- A player with a **broad external style** would, for example, focus on the entire field to assess the state of play.
- A coach could use a **broad internal style** to assess the whole game and then plan for the next game using his or her own judgements.
- A player would use a **narrow external style** to focus on a specific target, such as a golfer focusing on the hole before making a putt.
- A **narrow internal style** could be demonstrated by a player using mental rehearsal to concentrate on the feel of a shot or an aspect of play.

Some sports performers can concentrate on two streams of information at once and can switch from one attentive style to another quite easily. Such players are called **effective attenders**. A professional football player might use a broad style to scan the whole field to pick out an unmarked player to pass to and then switch to a narrow style to focus on hitting an accurate delivery. An **ineffective attender** would lose concentration easily and fail to cope with distractions.

To make sure that players are able to cope with distractions, coaches might conduct training sessions in front of a crowd so that the players become familiar with an audience. The ability to become an effective attender can be developed by experience. The coach could also practise the techniques of mental rehearsal and relaxation.

5   *Stress*

Stress is defined as the response of the body to demands or threats. Such threats in sport include the pressure of competition or concerns about not playing well. It is a performer's **perception** of stressful situations that determines whether the experience of stress is positive or negative. For example, at the start of a championship athletics race, the field is full of top-class runners:

- One athlete's recent efforts in training and her good form mean that she is looking forward to the race and cannot wait to test herself against the best. The positive feeling generated may help to improve performance and increase arousal and motivation to an appropriate level on the inverted-U graph.
- Another athlete feels that she will need to perform at her best to succeed and perhaps achieve a personal best time. She is worried about not doing well and the negative aspects of stress may induce anxiety that could hinder performance, causing tension and loss of concentration.

Figure 67 shows how the presence of a **stressor** causes a response from the body and results in either a positive or a negative experience.

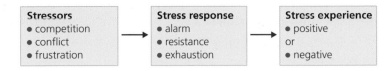

Figure 67

Stressors are defined as the changes in the sporting environment that cause stress and include:

- **conflict** (e.g. the threat of being marked by a skilled and physically strong player)
- **increased competition** (e.g. the grand final of a major cup competition)
- **frustrating circumstances** (e.g. being fouled or a poor refereeing decision)
- **physical changes** (e.g. the threat of playing extra time in a cup game causing fatigue or playing in hot conditions)
- the **crowd**, particularly if those watching you play are experts (e.g. a scout from a local club)

An initial shock at the presence of a stressor can cause alarm, which is then registered by the body through increases in heart rate, sweating and changes in adrenaline levels. If stressful symptoms persist, exhaustion may occur; however, the threat is usually overcome before such extremes happen.

6 Anxiety

Anxiety occurs when a performer views the threat of a stressor as negative and begins to worry. Irrational thinking and worrying about such things as not playing well, letting team mates down, recent injuries, meeting training demands or even personal off-field problems tend to cause muscular tension, lack of concentration, fear of failure and an inhibited performance. Such worries in sport can cause competitive anxiety or the fear of taking part in major events.

Some performers have a tendency to worry in most situations and are said to exhibit **trait anxiety** — they are born worriers who will always be concerned about performance and tend to view threats negatively all the time. **State anxiety** is a more temporary occurrence and relates to a specific situation, such as taking a penalty. The level of state anxiety can vary from moment to moment.

In sport, stress and anxiety are measured using the same methods as those used for evaluating personality traits, e.g. questionnaires, observation and physical measures such as the galvanic skin response (which records the level of sweat on the skin). One specific measure of stress is the **sports competition anxiety test** or SCAT, a questionnaire that assesses competitive anxiety. The results of the test were summarised by the psychologist Martens as follows:

- Performers are not equally anxious all the time. In training, a relaxed approach can be replaced by tension as an important game approaches.
- Levels of anxiety vary from near calm to almost complete panic in sport.
- A main cause of anxiety in sport is being watched by others whom we perceive to be experts. This perceived fear of being judged is called **evaluation apprehension**.

- Anxiety is a combination of trait and state effects. Those who have the anxiety trait are more likely to suffer state anxiety. A trait anxious hockey player would probably be even more nervous taking a penalty flick and could miss the opportunity to score.
- Anxiety is **multi-dimensional**, i.e. it has many facets, including physical effects, effects in the mind, the influence of confidence and the presence of trait and/or state anxieties.

6.1 A multi-dimensional approach to anxiety

The SCAT shows that anxiety has many facets:
- Anxiety in the mind, characterised by irrational thinking, fear of failure and lack of concentration, is called **cognitive anxiety**.
- Anxiety that is more physical and shows in bodily responses such as sweating, restlessness, increased heart rate, poor coordination and muscular tension is called **somatic anxiety**.

The relationship between cognitive anxiety and somatic anxiety is shown in Figures 68 and 69.

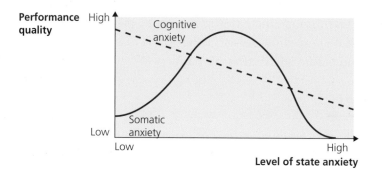

Figure 68

Figure 68 shows that somatic anxiety has a similar effect on performance as increased arousal does in the inverted-U theory. Increases in somatic anxiety can improve performance up to a point, after which further increases impair performance. However, cognitive anxiety has a negative linear effect, i.e. the greater the cognitive anxiety, the worse the performance. Figure 69 shows rises in somatic and cognitive anxiety in a performer before an event.

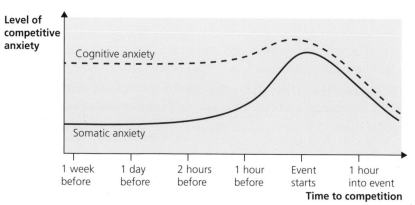

Figure 69

This shows that somatic anxiety tends to increase just before a competition or major game is due to begin and reduces as performance gets underway. Cognitive anxieties are present much earlier, and may be equally severe, despite the fact that the performer is not showing any physical signs of anxiety. The coach and player should therefore begin to control cognitive anxiety well before the game and introduce techniques to control somatic anxiety as the game approaches.

7 *Controlling stress and anxiety*

7.1 Controlling cognitive anxiety

Cognitive anxieties are controlled by various mental techniques:

- **Mental rehearsal** is when the performer goes over the actual physical requirements of the task in the mind without movement. The sequence of a dance routine could be rehearsed in the mind to ensure that the correct order is maintained.
- **Visualisation** involves picturing the techniques of a skill being practised on the training field as if competing for real. A football player practising free kicks could picture taking the same kick in a forthcoming game, noting the effects of the crowd, other players and the referee. The successful attempt in training is 'locked in' the player's thoughts so that it can be used in the real game.
- **Imagery** is an extension of these psychological techniques to include a mental recollection of a past success. This builds confidence and recreates the feelings of pride that were produced by that success. It is even possible for a performer to imagine an escape to help calm down and control any nerves, for example picturing himself or herself lying on a beach.
- **Positive self-talk** involves replacing any negative thoughts with positive ones. For example, the negative thought 'I'll never return her serve' is stopped and replaced with 'I can return her serve if I watch the ball'. Self-talk can also remind the performer of a technique or key element of the task. A rugby player taking a kick at goal may remind himself to aim for the left of the posts to allow the ball to be dragged in towards the target. Self-talk requires deep concentration.
- **Goal setting** can be used to lower cognitive anxieties, since the focus and concentration of the performer are improved.

Cognitive control techniques improve performance because they help to manage arousal, lower anxiety and provide motivation. Some research evidence suggests that mental processes activate muscle receptors, so that muscular stimulations occur without movement, providing more realistic practice than you might think. Players can use mental rehearsal to practise when injured, and cognitive control techniques can help experienced players concentrate on tactics and strategies.

7.2 Controlling somatic anxiety

Physical techniques are used to control somatic symptoms of stress and anxiety:

- **Relaxation methods** involve the performer tensing each muscle group and then gradually relaxing to feel a difference between the states of tension and relaxation (e.g. clenching the fists tightly and holding the tension for a few seconds before relaxing the grip). The performer must concentrate on tension reduction systematically.
- **Breathing control** can be used to lower anxiety (e.g. a hockey player taking deep breaths and reducing the rate of breathing before taking a penalty, in order to improve focus on the task). This is an attempt to redirect the anxiety away from the stressful situation.

- The technique of **biofeedback** is used to assess which method of relaxation is best for an individual. The performer is wired up to a heart rate monitor, for example, and then tries relaxation or cognitive methods to find out which lowers heart rate the most. However, taking part in an experiment may cause stress and render the results of this method unreliable.

7.3 Applying the techniques

It is important to include emotional control techniques, both somatic and cognitive, in your training programme, perhaps starting with short sessions and building up to **real time** (the actual time it takes you to do the task) as you become more competent. You should always focus on success. When you are in a game or performance situation, use some form of trigger or cue to help promote the mental processes. You could set goals for mental practice as well as physical practice, so that your progress is monitored. With practice, especially using the techniques of visualisation and imagery, you should be able to create vivid images.

8   *Social facilitation and social inhibition*

Social facilitation is defined as the behavioural effects of the presence of others. There is again a link between this concept and the inverted-U theory.

The inverted-U theory suggests that increased arousal can have differing effects on performance:
- If you are an expert, or the task being undertaken is simple, increased arousal can help performance.
- If you are a beginner, or the task is complex, lower arousal produces optimum performance and higher levels of arousal may cause performance to suffer.

The concepts of social facilitation and social inhibition support the inverted-U theory by stating that when we are being watched in sport, the main effect is to increase arousal levels; depending on the level of experience of the performer and the task in hand, there are two possible outcomes of being watched — you either play better (**facilitation**) or you play worse (**inhibition**).

When we play sport, there are four types of others who could be present:
- An **audience** just watches the performance, as the silent and appreciative crowd watching a snooker match would do.
- **Supporters** do not just watch; they become involved with the performance by cheering when things are going well or venting their displeasure when the team is not playing as well as they had hoped.
- **Co-actors** are present during performance, carrying out the same task at the same time but without any interference (e.g. a jogger on the other side of the road when someone is out on a run).
- **Competitors** are in direct conflict with the performer (e.g. the other athletes gathered at the start of a 100 m sprint).

While supporters and competitors can affect performance, the pure effects of others have been studied using an audience that simply watches.

Figure 70 outlines the concepts of social facilitation and social inhibition. As the diagram shows, another effect of being watched is to experience **evaluation apprehension**, or the fear of being judged. Players tend to think that the watching audience makes judgements on their performance and increased arousal and anxiety can result. This is particularly apparent if audience members are known to the player, or if experts on the game, such as a chief scout, are present.

The diagram also shows that at high arousal levels, we tend to pick out fewer cues and focus on the **dominant response**. There is a link here with drive theory, in that at high arousal the perceptual field narrows and only if the task is simple, or if the performer is an expert who can operate well on limited information, will it be possible for performance to be improved when being watched. Complex tasks that require more information to be dealt with could be impaired under conditions of high arousal in front of an audience — in other words, social inhibition occurs.

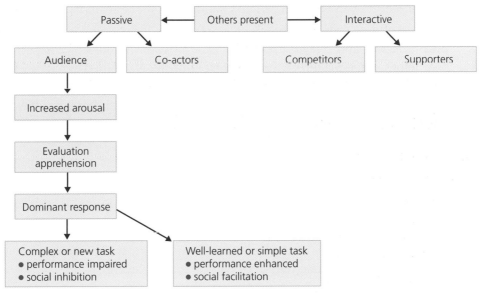

Figure 70

The influence of social facilitation can vary, depending on the situation. The **home field advantage** is the idea that most teams like to play in front of their own fans in their own stadium because it is more familiar and the support is positive. However, the increased expectancy of winning at home can produce added pressure and the effect of evaluation apprehension.

The **personality** of the performer can also influence social facilitation. Extroverts may respond more positively to a crowd and be more tolerant of increased adrenaline levels. Players with trait anxiety could suffer from the effects of being watched by a hostile crowd. A knowledgeable crowd could enhance the effect of evaluation apprehension, as the players might think that any judgements made would be meaningful. Previous experience of playing in front of a crowd may help to reduce anxiety — experienced professional players should be used to dealing with it.

8.1 Controlling social inhibition

To combat the distractive effects of an audience and to avoid social inhibition, both the coach and the player should become familiar with performing in front of a crowd by getting people to watch training sessions. The importance of the event should be reduced to relieve pressure — a coach might say to the players: 'It would be nice to qualify today but if we lose we can try again next week.' Relaxation techniques could be used to lower somatic anxiety; cognitive anxiety could be lowered by self-talk, imagery, mental rehearsal and visualisation. Ensuring that a performer can focus on the task and ignore the crowd is important, and the ability to concentrate can be developed in training.

9 | Attribution theory

The theory of attribution looks at the reasons we give for winning and losing in sport. These are important because they affect our future effort, motivation and behaviour.

Attribution is defined as the *perceived* cause of events or behaviour. When players lose a game, they tend to put the blame on something or someone else to protect their self-esteem. When players win, they give themselves credit for the success so that they can feel proud of their performance. Motivated players who play poorly may try harder next time round because their pride has been dented and they want to win back their self-respect.

Blaming others for losing and crediting ourselves for winning is known as **self-serving bias**. Coaches and players should be careful when accounting for performance, and bear in mind that the level of control the performer is deemed to have over the outcome of a sports event will affect future confidence and motivation. Coaches should provide reasons for a bad performance that can be addressed with fairly immediate effect, and should provide reasons for winning that can be maintained.

9.1 Reasons for performance

Internal reasons for a performance are those within a performer's control; reasons outside of a performer's control are said to be **external**. Changeable reasons are said to be **unstable**, while reasons that are not going to change in the short term are said to be **stable**.

Figure 71 represents a model for attribution in sport, which coaches can use after the event to give appropriate reasons for the result to players.

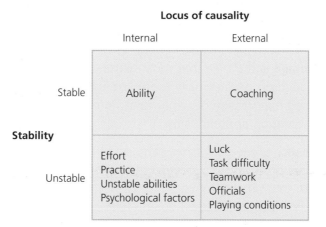

Figure 71

In order to maintain motivation, coaches should attribute the loss of a game to unstable and external reasons. They might blame:

- the referee for a bad decision
- bad luck, such as a shot striking a post instead of going into the net
- the fact that the competitors were a strong team

They might take a longer-term view and attribute a loss to coaching factors, indicating that a change of tactics is needed. They could suggest to players that some things might have to change before the next game, such as increasing the amount of practice and correcting some minor tactical faults, and encourage the whole team to put more effort into training and playing. Psychological factors, such as calming players down before the game so that less aggression is shown and fewer opportunities are given to the other team, could also be mentioned as something to change.

If the team won the game or played well, the result should be attributed to ability. Players should be praised for performing well and trying hard during the week or in the game. In this way, the coach is using the internal aspects of the attribution model to make the players continue to try hard in the future. High achievers in sport tend to attribute success internally. If players are shown a recording of their own performance, they tend to blame external reasons for their own failure but blame internal reasons for the failure of others, a phenomenon called the **observer-actor effect**.

9.2 Problems with attribution

Sometimes, the coach or player gets it wrong, and a lack of confidence can result from attributing failure to internal and stable reasons.

Being openly critical of a performer's ability may not be the most beneficial course of action. An athletics coach is likely to be more critical of a runner in the relay team who drops the baton due to lack of concentration than the incoming runner finishing last. If a player feels that a loss or a bad performance is consistently blamed on lack of ability, the phenomenon of **learned helplessness** can result. This can be **specific**, when the player thinks, 'the coach says I'm no good in midfield', or **global**, when the player begins to think 'I'm no good at sport'. This belief that failure is inevitable comes from blaming internal and stable reasons for losing.

To combat learned helplessness, the performer must be told that external and changeable reasons might be a more likely cause of failure than internal and stable ones, a tactic known as **attributional retraining**. The coach might suggest to the player, in a positive manner, that a change of tactics would be beneficial or that performance will improve sooner rather than later if the player continues to be matched against strong opponents. The player should get maximum encouragement from the coach and set goals that are achievable. Encouraging more effort in training under the guidance of a different coach may help, and coaches should stress that it is not necessarily the player's fault that losses have been more common than they would like.

Examiner's tip

It is common for exam questions to require you to relate theory to practice by including an example in your answer. Sometimes the example will relate to a specific sport, for example: 'As a coach of team players, how would you ensure that your team does not suffer from social inhibition?' Whenever questions ask you to imagine you are a *team* coach, make sure that you do not give an example from an *individual* sport, such as athletics.

You may have noticed a common thread running through all the concepts related to emotional control — the relationship between arousal and performance. You should make sure that you know this theory thoroughly, as it can be used in most answers and will gain you marks. Arousal is a major topic, and the methods used to control it are common to most questions. Concepts such as mental rehearsal, visualisation, imagery, relaxation techniques and positive self-talk can be used to control arousal, raise confidence, deal with the distractions of a crowd and make sure that motivation is maintained. There is therefore a 'pool' of information you could use to gain marks in different questions, saving you valuable revision time.

Section 3
Sociocultural & historical studies

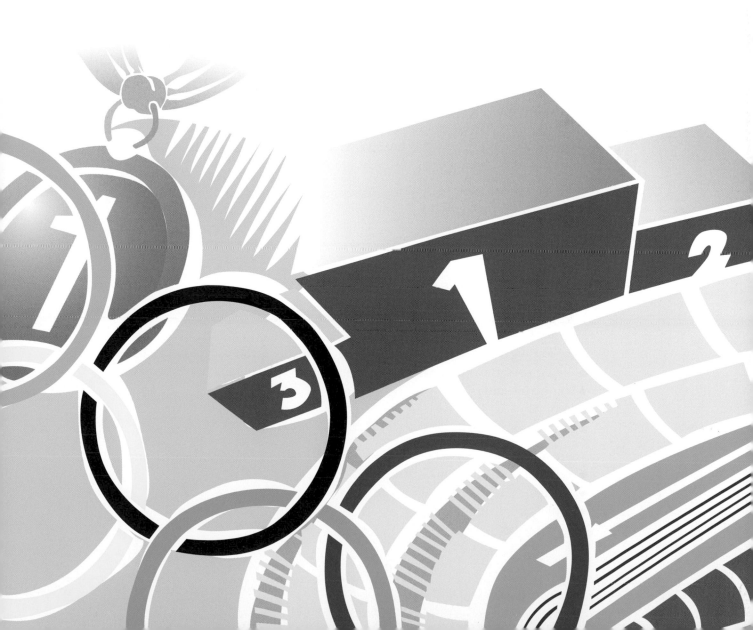

Concepts in sport and PE

By the end of this topic, you should:
● know the key characteristics and functions/values of a range of concepts, including leisure, play, physical recreation, physical education, outdoor and adventurous activities (OAA), and sport
● understand how active leisure links to physical recreation
● be able to identify the value of such concepts to individuals and society

1 Physical education

Physical education (PE) can be defined as a formally planned and taught curriculum, designed to increase knowledge and values through physical activity and experience. In the UK, it is delivered through a structure known as the National Curriculum. PE can be viewed as a triangular model, as shown in Figure 72.

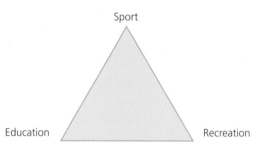

Figure 72

The three elements of this model are defined as follows:
● **education** — PE as a compulsory curriculum subject/taught in lessons
● **sport** — organised, optional extra-curricular activities of a competitive nature
● **recreation** — activities freely engaged in by pupils in extra-curricular time with an emphasis on participation as opposed to results

The main objective of PE is to increase pupils' knowledge of:
● health and fitness
● motor skills/physical skills
● tactics/decision making
● different roles (e.g. performer/coach/official)
● how to be a successful leader
● how to be active in leisure time and achieve lifelong involvement in physical activity

PE promotes values such as:
● becoming a civilised member of society (**social control**)
● being able to work in a team/cooperate
● caring for others
● morality
● a sense of fair play

There are six areas of activity in National Curriculum PE at Key Stages 1 and 2:
● outdoor and adventurous activities
● games
● athletics
● gymnastics

- dance
- swimming

From 2008, changes to the National Curriculum allow teachers of Key Stages 3 and 4 more autonomy, so they can deliver the various aims of the curriculum without restrictions as to which areas of activity they cover. There is also a focus on more complex skill development as children progress. Increased prominence is given to fitness and exercise activities, linked to promotion of the government's health agenda.

You should be able to reflect on your own National Curriculum, lesson-time PE experiences and link these, with practical examples, to the definition and features identified above. For example, gymnastics is likely to involve:

- developing fitness (e.g. flexibility)
- working together in a group to solve a set task
- showing concern for someone who is anxious in a lesson
- trusting someone to support you in a balance

2 Outdoor and adventurous activities (OAA)

Outdoor and adventurous activities (OAA) are one of the six areas of National Curriculum PE and can be defined as the achievement of educational objectives via guided and direct experiences in the natural environment. Such activities have many purposes/functions, including a role in heightening awareness of, and respect for:

- others — working in a group, developing team, social and communication skills
- oneself — through meeting challenges (self-discovery/self-realisation/self-esteem)
- the environment — respect for the countryside/aesthetic appreciation
- danger/risk/safety

Factors that may negatively affect a pupil's OAA experience include:

- staffing — lack of training, experience, qualifications, motivation
- time — lack of time, travel often involved
- money/resources — too expensive for schools and parents, lack of equipment
- danger — parents and teachers may be deterred from certain activities that are inherently dangerous (e.g. skiing)

3 Leisure

Leisure can be defined as any spare time in life when there is an opportunity for choice, as all obligations have been met. Leisure time should be an opportunity for individuals to have fun and enjoy themselves.

Leisure can serve many functions/purposes. For an individual, leisure can provide:

- **relaxation**, unwinding/de-stressing from work
- opportunity to **socialise** and meet people
- improvements in **health** and **fitness**

For society, local authorities and the government, leisure can:

- encourage **conformity**/civilised society/social control
- improve **health and wellbeing**/decrease strain on the National Health Service
- encourage social and racial mixing/**integration** of society

A number of factors can affect a person's participation in active leisure, including:

- **socioeconomic status** — money and time available may restrict access
- **gender** — perceptions about what is masculine and feminine may affect the activities or clubs available (e.g. a lack of dance groups for men and boxing clubs for women)
- **ethnicity** — cultural and religious observances may affect opportunities to participate in leisure activities
- **disability** — access to and availability of sports facilities/clubs/coaches may be restricted
- **age** — retired people have more time, but may have less money or poorer health

3.1 Links between leisure and recreation

Physical recreation can be defined as the active aspect of leisure. Recreation is entered into voluntarily during free time and people choose which activities they take part in. It focuses on participation as opposed to results, providing benefits to an individual and to society that are similar to those of leisure. The values/purposes of recreation include allowing individuals to:

- relax and unwind
- be creative and do something they are proud of (self-fulfillment/self-realisation/self-esteem)
- socialise and meet new people
- improve health and fitness/decrease strain on the NHS (important to an individual as well as society in general)
- improve morality and increase conformity/social control — a socially civilising force (e.g. used in inner-city crime-reduction schemes among young offenders)

As with leisure, an individual's choice of recreation activities is influenced by a number of different factors including socioeconomic status, gender, age and ethnicity. Sometimes, more than one factor applies to an individual, making it difficult for him or her to take part in a healthy physical activity in his or her spare time. For example, if you are 60, female, disabled and of ethnic minority status, you are less likely to participate in recreation than a younger, able-bodied, white male.

3.2 OAA as outdoor recreation

Outdoor recreation can be defined as physical activity pursued in free time in the natural environment, which includes a sense of risk and adventure:

- **Real risk** actually exists; experienced performers sometimes participate in activities such as rock-climbing with no safety harness for the extra adrenaline rush this gives them.
- **Perceived risk** is in a person's head only; the situation is safe due to precautions or expert instruction, which minimise the element of danger for inexperienced performers but still allow the *sense* of risk.

Popular examples of OAA activities include rock-climbing, mountain walking and canoeing. This type of recreation serves a number of different purposes for people, including:

- **relaxation** — allowing you to unwind from everyday life and providing an alternative experience

- personal **challenge** — allowing personal limits to be reached and providing self-realisation and self-fulfilment; conquering fears (e.g. of heights)
- aesthetic **appreciation of the natural environment** and countryside
- working in a **team** — cooperating to achieve a set task or common goal
- developing **leadership** skills
- developing **survival** skills

4 Play

As a concept, play can be characterised by the following attributes. It is:
- **fun** — designed for enjoyment, a non-serious activity
- **childlike**, innocent and simple
- **spontaneous** — spur of the moment/you can start or change as you wish
- **flexible** — rules and time boundaries are not fixed
- **self-administered** — those playing determine the rules and time for play/self-officiate

It is important to understand the different functions/values of play, particularly for a child but also for an adult.

The functions/values of play for a child fall into four categories:
- **social** — development of social skills and practice for future social roles
- **cognitive** — decision-making and learning to control emotions
- **physical** — children become active and improve their health, fitness and coordination
- **moral** — fair play/learning to share

The main functions/values of play for an adult are based on psychological benefits. Play provides:
- stress relief
- an escape from reality
- recuperation from daily duties
- an opportunity to relax

5 Sport

Sport can be defined as a contrived competitive experience. The key values/objectives and characteristics of sport include:
- **competitiveness** — the will to win
- **seriousness** — the need to win at all costs, particularly at professional/elite levels
- **strict rule structures** — administered by national governing bodies
- **commitment to training** — a high level of fitness and skill is required
- importance of **extrinsic rewards**, for example medals, trophies or money
- an element of **chance or luck**

It is important to note that the values of sport to individuals and society are similar to those stated above in relation to active leisure/physical recreation.

Examiner's tip

An understanding of this topic is required at AS by all the exam boards. Questions may either require a separate consideration of the concepts (i.e. definitions, key characteristics and functions) or involve comparing and contrasting them. You might have to state the shared characteristics of play and recreation, or explain how an activity such as swimming can be educational, recreational and sporting. It is therefore important to understand all the key concepts and be able to apply them to practical examples.

You should aim to make a variety of relevant points in your answers. Unless the question asks for a certain number, make more points than there are marks available, to ensure that you gain the maximum allocation. OCR AS Unit G451 no longer requires a consideration of play, so you do not need to revise it if you are following this specification.

TOPIC 2 Government policies on school sport and PE

By the end of this topic, you should:

- know the key features of current initiatives in school sport, e.g. the government's sports strategy/PESSCL
- know what a sports college is and be able to outline its functions and benefits
- be able to identify the roles of various national agencies, e.g. the Youth Sport Trust
- be able to explain what school sport coordinators (SSCos) are and outline their main functions

1 Sports strategy: key features

The key features of the government's sports strategy are:

- the introduction of school sport coordinators (SSCos)
- an increase in the quantity of school and community sports facilities
- an increase in the quality and quantity of available coaches (including the 'Coaching for Teachers' scheme coordinated through Sports Coach UK)
- protection of school playing fields
- improved links between schools and elite performers (visits by 'world-class' lottery-funded sports performers/Sport England's 'Sporting Champions')
- increased numbers of sports colleges offering specialist education for sport
- awards for good practice in school sport/PE provision (e.g. extra-curricular provision/links between schools/local sports clubs/PESSCL and sharing facilities/coaches etc.)

1.1 Sports colleges

A sports college is a secondary school, teaching pupils aged 11–16 or 11–18, with a specialist status for sport. As part of the government's specialist schools programme, its key features and benefits include:

- innovative curriculum design (its pioneering teaching and learning ideas are shared with other schools as examples of good practice)
- improved links to primary schools and community sports organisations
- work with the national governing bodies (NGBs) of sport to support the development of talented youngsters
- improved status and funding
- excellent facilities and coaching
- increased curricular and extracurricular time/opportunities for sport/PE
- a wider variety of sports on offer (increased breadth)
- potential for improved student motivation and better exam performance
- peer group support
- competition among like-minded individuals to develop excellence

1.2 National agencies promoting school sport/PE

There are various national agencies that support the promotion and development of sporting activity for school children. An example is the **Youth Sport Trust**, which has been given responsibility for raising standards in school PE/sport through its own initiatives as well as coordinating the work of other organisations involved with school-aged children.

The Youth Sport Trust:

- brings sport to life for young people
- runs the TOP schemes (e.g. TOP Play/TOP Sport)
- trains leaders in sport and recreation (e.g. Step into Sport)
- aims to improve the quality of teaching and coaching (e.g. via resources and session plans as part of TOP Sport for 7–11-year-olds)
- promotes the benefits of sport to youngsters (e.g. via a 'School Sport Champion' — Dame Kelly Holmes served in this role in 2007 and beyond)

1.3 School sports coordinators (SSCos)

School sports coordinators are individuals who seek to improve the quality and quantity of after-school sport and inter-school competition. They are of key importance in increasing access to sport for disadvantaged young people. They also provide PE and sports courses for teachers and other young adults for ongoing professional development.

Examiner's tip

At AS, all the exam boards require an understanding of current government policies and initiatives for school PE. Questions on the benefits of sports college status are popular at AS and should be considered in relation to students attending sports colleges as well as the wider community they serve. Knowledge of various national sports bodies and their initiatives is useful here — a number of examiner reports comment on candidates' 'lack of knowledge of relevant school sports initiatives'. You could supplement your revision of these initiatives by using the internet. Sport England and the Youth Sport Trust both have informative websites that will keep you up to date with the latest initiatives and allow you to impress the examiners:

- **www.sportengland.org**
- **www.youthsporttrust.org**

3 Development of sports excellence in the UK

By the end of this topic, you should:

- know what is meant by excellence and elitism
- be able to identify a number of initiatives for excellence in the UK and explain how they are funded
- be able to identify some key organisations, and their main functions in relation to excellence
- understand the problems associated with the pursuit of excellence
- recognise key characteristics of world games and reasons for investing in hosting global sports events

1 Excellence and elitism

Excellence is found at the top of the sports development pyramid and can be defined as the standard of the best or highly proficient performers. Elitism is the term used to describe the focus of resources on top performers (e.g. money, specialist facilities and top-level coaching). There are various initiatives and policies in the UK designed to improve top-level performance standards, including:

- **schools of excellence** and **academies** for elite performers
- **sports colleges** that focus on particular sports and have links with the UK Sports Institute or national governing bodies (NGBs) (e.g. Burleigh Sports College focuses on tennis and has links to Loughborough University and the Lawn Tennis Association)
- **funding** through the National Lottery and/or the World Class Performance Programme, the Talented Athlete Scholarship Scheme (TASS, and TASS 2012), scholarships, sponsorship deals, SportsAid and other sources
- the **United Kingdom Sports Institute** (UKSI)/home country institutes of sport (e.g. English Institute of Sport, EIS), a network of centres throughout the UK providing specialist facilities, top-level coaching, specialist medical advice, sports science support and performance lifestyle advice for top-level performers
- **professional coaching policies**, such as those operated by Sports Coach UK and NGBs of sport

The functions of organisations involved in the development of excellence are outlined below.

Key organisations	Functions
Sport England	Aims for 'more medals' via distribution of lottery funding; World Class programme
UK Sport	Focus on elite performers; key role in running of UKSI
Sports Coach UK	Development of professional coaching policies; coach education schemes; coaching for teachers
NGBs	Sports-specific developments; talent identification schemes

1.1 Problems associated with excellence

- **Inadequate funding** — particularly apparent when the UK is compared with other countries, such as Australia.
- **Disproportionate funding** — governments must balance the amount spent on sport with money needed for other key areas such as health or education. Spending on the

London 2012 Olympic Games has received criticism because billions of pounds are being diverted from other good causes in society and mass participation initiatives in sport.

- **Lack of availability** of top-level coaches and specialist facilities to develop top-level performers to their full potential (e.g. 50 m indoor swimming pools).
- **Focus on certain sports** — less popular sports may be neglected or have funding taken back if they fail to meet performance targets under UK Sport's 'no compromise' approach to elite sports funding (e.g. gymnastics and hockey).
- Tradition of **non-government intervention** at the top level of sport (i.e. **autonomy**).

2 World games

World games:

- involve **elite-level performers** (the aim being to decide the number 1 performer in the world for a specific activity)
- can be **multi-sport** (Olympics) or **single-sport** (football World Cup)
- constitute a **national showpiece**
- are **commercialised** and attract **world-wide media coverage**
- can help **integrate nations**
- may be associated with **deviancy** and **cheating** (e.g. taking drugs)

Billions of pounds are invested in hosting elite sporting events, such as the London 2012 Olympic Games. Reasons for this include several benefits for the host country:

- international **promotion** of a city or country
- improved **infrastructure** (e.g. roads, railways and airports)
- increased **national pride** ('feel-good' factor)
- **economic benefits** and **regeneration**
- boost to **participation** and the **health and fitness** of the nation

Advantages are also evident for individuals:

- opportunity to **represent country** on home soil at the highest level
- chance to gain **extrinsic** rewards and **sponsorship** opportunities
- opportunity to be **officially recognised as the number one performer** in the world in a specific activity

Examiner's tip

All the exam boards require knowledge of policies and initiatives designed to improve elite-level performance in the UK. Edexcel Units 1 and 3, OCR Unit G451 and AQA Unit 3 expect sound knowledge of this ever-developing topic. Keep an eye on the news media, as elite-level performance receives a good deal of publicity. Questions may relate generally to key initiatives designed to improve sporting excellence in the UK or may ask about the specific roles of various organisations such as UK Sport or NGBs.

AQA Unit 3 requires knowledge of characteristics of world games. OCR Unit G451 and AQA Unit 3 expect you to know reasons for investing resources in elite sporting events.

4 Target groups

By the end of this topic, you should:
- know what target groups are and be able to give examples
- know the effects of gender on participation and progression in sport and be able to explain how problems can be overcome
- be able to outline the causes of, and possible solutions for, the under-representation of the disabled, ethnic minorities and the elderly in sport and recreation
- be able to consider whether social class is still an issue in sporting participation in twenty-first-century Britain

1 Definition

According to organisations such as Sport England, a target group is a group or section of society that is under-represented in sport and recreation in relation to its presence in society as a whole. Examples of target groups include:
- women
- ethnic minorities
- the disabled
- the elderly

Social class may also affect participation in physical activity in modern-day society.

2 Women

2.1 Barrriers to women's participation

Women's participation in physical activity is affected by a variety of different barriers, such as:
- lack of time — many women have family/work commitments and domestic responsibilities
- lack of competitions/leagues — this makes participation and professionalism more difficult
- restricted choice of activities/clubs to attend (e.g. at leisure centres/in school PE programmes)
- limited career opportunities (e.g. there are fewer female coaches/administrators than male, particularly in elite-level sport)
- lower rewards and prize money
- fewer sponsorship opportunities
- less disposable income available for sport or recreation
- fewer role models to aspire to
- less media coverage of women's sports (often deemed to be less exciting than those of their male counterparts)
- tradition/stereotypes — many activities are perceived as being exclusively for men (e.g. boxing and rugby)
- lack of self-confidence

2.2 Improvement in women's participation

It is important to increase women's participation in sport for several reasons:

- to improve health and fitness
- to help with weight control
- to help improve self-esteem
- to improve social/teamwork skills

Visit **www.whatworksforwomen.org.uk** for examples of initiatives that have been successful in raising female participation in physical activity.

Possible solutions and reasons for improvements so far include:

- a wider range of activities on offer
- more clubs and leagues
- positive discrimination
- women-only sessions at local leisure centres
- greater financial independence (more women working, with their own disposable income)
- reduced entry rates or fees (e.g. to leisure centres and clubs)
- greater provision of crèches/childcare in leisure centres to decrease the problems associated with domestic responsibilities
- more media coverage/promotions/campaigns (e.g. women's World Cup from China in 2007 on BBC television)
- more positive role models (e.g. Paula Radcliffe)
- more diversity — a wider range of activities on offer for girls in National Curriculum PE (e.g. girls' soccer/rugby)

3 *Disability*

Disabilities are categorised in the following ways for sporting competition:

- physical
- mental/learning difficulties
- sensory impairment (e.g. blindness/deafness)
- cerebral palsy
- transplant patients

People with a disability are under-represented in sport for a variety of reasons, including:

- limited career opportunities — there are few disabled coaches or administrators
- lack of competitive opportunities, clubs or leagues
- restricted choice of activities
- lack of appropriate transport, space, equipment and facilities
- poor accessibility to/within sports facilities
- lack of confidence/negative self-image
- fewer role models
- lack of media coverage
- myths about participation in sport, i.e. that it may be dangerous or damaging to health

Possible solutions include:

- training of more disabled coaches and provision of specialist coaching
- more competitive opportunities, clubs and leagues
- adaptation of sports as appropriate (e.g. wheelchair basketball)
- improved accessibility to/within sports facilities

- media coverage of role models (e.g. Special Olympians/Paralympics)
- promotions and campaigns (e.g. by Sport England/Disability Sport England)
- increased awareness/education (e.g. to dispel myths)

4 Ethnic minorities

This is a popular exam topic. You should be familiar with the ways in which a person's ethnic background may influence his or her participation in sport and recreation.

Reasons for the under-representation of ethnic minorities include:
- racial discrimination — threats or abuse deterring participation
- certain cultural groups valuing education, careers or religious duties as more important than sport and recreation
- some values of sport conflicting with religious observances
- fewer role models in certain sports
- low self-esteem and fear of rejection
- ethnic stereotyping affecting an individual's choice of sport

Possible solutions include:
- tougher laws against, and harsher punishments for, racist abuse by performers or spectators
- positive use of ethnic minority role models
- increased media coverage
- teacher and coach education on the effects of stereotyping
- sport-led campaigns such as 'Kick it out' in football

The term '**stacking**' refers to the disproportionate concentration of ethnic minority players in certain positions in a sports team, which tends to be based on the stereotyped view that they are best suited to roles that require physical ability, rather than decision-making or communication skills. For example, there are a disproportionate number of ethnic minority centre forwards in football, a position that depends on explosive speed rather than decision-making.

5 The elderly

Reasons for the lack of involvement of elderly people in sport or recreation include:
- lack of money
- transport difficulties
- low self-esteem
- fewer role models
- lack of specialist coaches

Possible solutions include:
- specialist clubs for the elderly
- reduced entry fees to leisure centres
- training specialist coaches to work with the elderly

6 Social class

You may be asked to consider whether social class has an impact on participation in physical activity in the UK today. You could consider issues of:

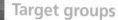
- lower income
- lower levels of self-esteem
- lack of motivation to exercise

There are still sports with 'working-class' links, such as rugby league and darts. Those more associated with the 'middle classes' and 'upper classes' include hockey and horse riding. However, increased equality in society means the vast majority of sports activities are available to all, even if there is an obvious social-class bias in some.

Examiner's tip

An understanding of the various target groups identified by Sport England as being under-represented in sport or recreation is important to all exam boards at AS. You must be able to identify the different causes of under-representation as well as possible solutions.

The different exam boards have identified similar target groups to study, but key differences are that the elderly are not mentioned on the AQA specification and OCR makes no reference to social class.

Questions on women, ethnic minorities and people with disabilities are popular and occur on a regular basis. Unless the question states otherwise, make more points than there are marks available; examiner mark schemes award only 1 mark for a number of similar points (e.g. role models/media coverage).

You should be clear about the differences between opportunity (the chance), provision (the facilities, coaches etc.) and esteem (self-confidence/belief), particularly if you are following OCR Unit G451.

5 The sports development pyramid/key organisations

By the end of this topic, you should be able to:
- draw the sports development pyramid and identify/explain the different levels
- list examples of key organisations involved in setting sports policies in the UK
- identify the functions of these organisations

1 The sports development pyramid

The sports development pyramid is a way of categorising the different levels of involvement in sport and physical activity. In the UK, it has a wide base and becomes smaller in width and numbers as the top of the pyramid is reached.

The levels of the pyramid from top to bottom are:
- **excellence** — elite performance standards, highest skill levels
- **performance** — taking part with a commitment to regular competitive involvement and improvement of performance
- **participation** — regular recreation for fun/social/health and fitness purposes
- **foundation** — first introduction to sport or PE/grass roots/primary school PE

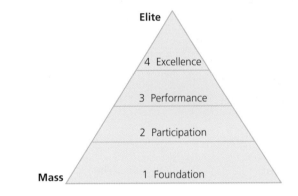

Figure 73

2 Key organisations

There are various organisations involved in raising levels of participation and standards of performance in sport, and they are responsible for devising and implementing sports policies at all levels of the pyramid. You need to know their precise functions and be able to give examples of their initiatives. Organisations in the UK include:
- home country sports councils (e.g. Sport England)
- UK Sport
- the Youth Sport Trust
- Sports Coach UK
- national governing bodies (e.g. England Netball, Football Association (FA), UK Athletics)
- Disability Sport England
- Women's Sport Foundation

The key functions of these organisations are outlined in the table below.

Key organisation	Initiatives for mass participation	Initiatives for excellence
Sport England	● Responsibility for raising participation in community sport ● 'Start, stay and succeed' and Get Active — Active Communities/Active Places/Sport Action Zones ● National Lottery funding of facilities ● Awards for All ● Sporting Champions (visits to schools by elite lottery-funded athletes acting as positive role models for participation)	
UK Sport		● National Lottery funding for top-level performers ● World Class Performance Programme ● Supporting high-performance sport/attracting major sports events to the UK ● Responsibility for doping control and testing in UK/100% ME programme ● Overseeing the United Kingdom Sports Institute (UKSI)
Youth Sport Trust	● Responsibility for school PE/sport ● TOPs programmes (e.g. TOP Sport for 7–11-year-olds) ● Training teachers/sports leaders for TOPs/Step into Sport ● Providing resources (e.g. TOP kitbags) ● Appointing a School Sport Champion (e.g. Dame Kelly Holmes) ● Sky Living for Sport — developed in England in 2007 with Darren Campbell as one of its ambassadors	
Sports Coach UK	● Working to improve the quality of coaching at mass-participation level ● Responsibility for the Coaching for Teachers initiative	● High Performance Coaching development

Key organisation	Initiatives for mass participation	Initiatives for excellence
National Governing Bodies (NGBs)	• Examples include the High 5 netball initiative run by England Netball and Sports Hall Athletics by UK Athletics	• Working to improve the quality of coaching at elite level • Examples include the proposed FA National Soccer Centre in Burton-on-Trent, which gained renewed support following England's failure to qualify for Euro 2008 • Organising regional and national competitions to help the progress of performance standards
Disability Sport England (DSE)	• Catering for all forms of disability at all levels of participation • Educating society on the needs/capabilities of disabled sports performers	
Women's Sport Foundation (WSF)	• Examples include launching and developing a national action plan for women's and girls' sport • New website **www.what worksforwomen.org.uk** to promote schemes that have improved participation levels among women	• Examples include a campaign to increase the numbers of women in high-performance coaching

2.1 British Olympic Association (BOA)

The British Olympic Association is a non-government organisation that aims to:

- encourage interest in the Olympic Games
- foster the ideals of the Olympic movement
- organise and coordinate British participation in the Olympics
- assist the NGBs in their preparation for competitions (e.g. setting up a 'performance unit' for elite-level athletes)

Examiner's tip

For OCR Unit G451, AQA Units 1 and 3 and Edexcel Units 1 and 3, you must have an understanding of a number of key sports policy organisations and the initiatives they are responsible for implementing. Specific questions are often set on the functions of key bodies such as UK Sport and the home country sports councils (e.g. Sport England), while knowledge of initiatives they are involved in may be related to more general questions on excellence or mass participation.

Some questions may address the sports development pyramid; these require the use of precise terminology in order to make your understanding of its different levels clear to the examiner.

6 Organisation and funding of sport in the UK

By the end of this topic, you should:
- be able to identify sources of funding for sport in the UK, including public, private and voluntary sources
- know the differences between private, public and voluntary local sport organisations
- know what is meant by 'Best Value'

1 Background to funding

There is a diverse range of funding available for sports performers and recreation provision in the UK. When compared with countries such as Australia and France, public spending on sport has traditionally been limited, although the introduction of National Lottery money into the sports arena has had a positive impact on funding at all levels. Private funding, in the form of sponsorship, tends to be directed towards elite and professional performers, as sponsors wish to exploit the commercial and media opportunities this presents. However, sport in the UK has a tradition of autonomy — national governing bodies and voluntary clubs wish to retain the power to make their own decisions, and this may have inhibited funding developments. Voluntary funds can be received from sources such as parents and family wishing to support a talented performer financially in his or her development.

2 Funding

Funding for sport in the UK can be gained from a variety of sources. These can be:
- **public** (e.g. central government, local authorities)
- **private** (e.g. businesses, individual sponsorship)
- **voluntary** (e.g. individuals or clubs funding their own training and participation, perhaps by fundraising or paying/charging membership fees)

3 Organisations

Organisations involved in sport and recreation can be divided into three groups: **public sector**, **private sector** and **voluntary sector**.

Public-sector groups:
- are owned by the local authority (i.e. by rate-payers)
- trade on a profit-and-loss basis
- have a duty to provide high-quality recreational services
- promote mass participation

Private-sector groups:
- are privately owned businesses or registered companies
- promote activities that bring profits rather than seeking to promote mass participation
- offer high-quality service to members who pay a fee

Voluntary-sector groups:
- are owned by members on a trust basis
- are managed by members on a voluntary basis
- trade on a break-even basis
- may need to increase membership to raise funds, but often focus on attracting better performers to improve chances of winning

4 Best Value

The government introduced the policy of 'Best Value' in an attempt to improve the quality of sport and recreation provision by local authorities. Some of its main features include:

- trying to get the best value for money
- giving the best-value experience possible
- finding out what the public or community wants
- setting standards
- delivering services to match standards
- measuring success
- reviewing expectations

Examiner's tip

OCR Unit G451 and AQA Unit 1 require broad knowledge of the organisation and funding of sport in the UK at local and national levels. Questions either focus on a specific aspect, such as the meaning of 'Best Value', or require a more critical insight into how the UK organises and funds its sport, perhaps focusing on government investment in sport and recreation in comparison with other demands of society (e.g. health care and education).

Candidates' answers often lack in-depth critical understanding of funding and policy provision in the different sectors. This does not tend to be a problem in simple factual-recall questions (e.g. 'Define what is meant by "public-sector sport/recreation"') but is more crucial when answering questions that offer a larger number of marks and require more detailed and well-planned responses (e.g. comparing sectors/discussing their advantages and disadvantages).

TOPIC 7 Ethical behaviour and legal issues

By the end of this topic, you should:
- know the meaning of key terms to do with sporting ethics
- be able to list the causes of, and possible solutions to, the problems of performer violence, the use of performance-enhancing drugs in sport and dysfunctional spectator behaviour
- understand why the law has become increasingly involved with modern-day sport
- be aware of technological developments in sport and their impact on performers/spectators (e.g. Hawk-Eye)

1 Definitions

Sportsmanship is playing according to the spirit of fair play and within the rules and etiquette (unwritten rules) of the game. Examples include shaking hands with the opposition at the end of a contest and applauding an opponent's excellent play. This links to the Olympic Oath and Olympic ideal, which maintain that participation in the Olympics should be within the 'true spirit of sportsmanship'. Sportsmanship allows the game to run smoothly and promotes goodwill among players and spectators.

Gamesmanship is using unfair practices to gain an advantage, often stretching the rules and etiquette of the game to their absolute limits. Examples would be time wasting or sledging opponents (deliberately using verbal abuse for psychological gain). In the Australia vs India test match cricket series at the start of 2008, there were accusations from both sides and threats to withdraw from the series by India. Gamesmanship leads to disruptions in play and trouble between players and between spectators.

The '**contract to compete**' is a mutual agreement to play fairly according to the rules of the sport. If a player fails to keep this agreement, for example by using drugs or taking bribes, the competition is no longer fair and the contract is broken.

2 Performer violence

Performer violence can be defined as any aggressive act by a performer outside the rules of sport. Examples include:
- high tackling (rugby/football)
- head-butting (football)
- ear-biting (boxing)

The causes of performer violence include:
- a 'win at all costs' attitude
- frustration with the referee, opponents, team mates or the crowd
- the attitude of the coach or team mates if they encourage violent acts
- local rivalry with the opposition
- the importance of the result
- receiving physical or verbal abuse (retaliation)
- high rewards of winning

Possible solutions to the problem include:
- the use of video technology or a panel to assess and adjudicate on unfair play; this is increasingly used in modern-day sport, especially rugby league and rugby union
- more severe penalties (e.g. bans, fines or 'sin bins')

- education and an emphasis on the ethos of fair play; UK Sport promotes ethically fair sport as part of its 100% ME programme

3 Performance-enhancing drugs

Some examples of performance-enhancing drugs and their effects are:
- diuretics — weight loss as a result of fluid loss
- narcotic analgesics — pain reduction or masking of an injury
- beta blockers — relaxing effect/calming
- EPO — increased endurance

There are various reasons why performers may be tempted to use drugs, including:
- the potential for improving physical performance and therefore increasing the chance of winning
- pressure from coaches and/or peers
- a 'win at all costs' attitude fostered by the prospect of high rewards (e.g. money and fame)
- the belief that everybody else is doing it (it 'levels the playing field')
- a lack of deterrents or a perceived low risk of being caught

Clearly, there are strong reasons against the use of drugs in sport, particularly that:
- it is illegal
- it is immoral — it gives an unfair advantage and is therefore a form of cheating
- it lowers the status of the sport
- it provides a poor example to youngsters
- there are associated health problems, such as addiction, heart disease and excessive aggression

Possible solutions to the problem include:
- stricter, more rigorous testing carried out at random
- stricter deterrents and punishments (e.g. life-long bans or imprisonment, as was the case for disgraced American sprinter Marion Jones)
- coordinated education programmes for athletes and coaches, which highlight the health and moral issues (e.g. UK Sport's 100% ME programme)
- use of positive role models to reinforce the anti-drugs message (e.g. Paula Radcliffe)

However, there are difficulties with the implementation of these solutions:
- the testing system may be inaccurate, particularly where masking agents are used
- drugs may be used legally for medical reasons
- widespread and improved testing is costly
- access to performers may be difficult
- performers are prepared to take the risk as the rewards are so high

There is also a dubious '**counter-culture**' argument proposing the legalisation of drugs in sport because of the expense of drugs testing, ineffective testing, the increase in performance standards possible from drug taking which crowds want to see and the fact that money spent on drugs testing could be spent better elsewhere.

4 Dysfunctional spectator behaviour

Dysfunctional spectator behaviour is violence and the intent to harm others. A key example is **football hooliganism**.

Causes of football hooliganism include:
- consumption of alcohol
- violence by performers on the field of play
- pre-match 'hype' increased by media coverage (e.g. in tabloid newspapers)
- poor refereeing
- behaviour of opposition fans (e.g. abusive chants)
- an unfavourable score or result (i.e. your team is losing)
- religious or partisan differences (e.g. Celtic vs Rangers)
- diminished individual responsibility as part of a crowd

Some solutions to the problem include:
- the use of CCTV
- improved policing and security
- tougher deterrents
- control of alcohol sales
- changing kick-off times to earlier in the day to reduce alcohol consumption (e.g. when local derbies/matches with strong rivalries are played)
- provision of family enclosures to encourage a family atmosphere
- membership schemes to control entrance to the stadium

5 *Sport and the law*

In recent years, sport and the law have become inextricably linked. Litigation (i.e. taking legal action) has been increasingly used to:
- eliminate discrimination (e.g. racist chanting is against the law)
- pursue rights attained by civil law (e.g. Brian McCord was the first player to win damages against another player and his club when he received £250,000 for a career-ending tackle in 1993, and many other cases have followed this lead)
- try to eliminate drug cheats (e.g. Marion Jones was sent to jail in the USA for perjury early in 2008)
- allow footballers to pursue freedom of contract following the Bosman ruling

6 *Sports technology: Hawk-Eye*

One high-profile example of the use of technology in modern-day sport is Hawk-Eye — a computer linked to 10 on-court cameras that makes a billion calculations on every point in order to rule on line calls. It has been used by Channel 4 in its cricket coverage since 2001 and was introduced at the Wimbledon tennis championships in 2007.

Most players, officials and spectators support its use, as it takes the sting out of contentious line calls and provides an extra element of drama as everyone awaits the computer's verdict. However, some complaints are raised about its reliability and the fact that sometimes it gets overused/misused; for example at the end of sets, players can take advantage of the situation to challenge a call and get more of a breather — a form of gamesmanship.

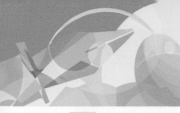

Examiner's tip

Deviance, sporting ethics and spectator behaviour are key topics for all the major exam boards. They relate particularly to elite-level sport in modern-day society, and feature prominently as important issues on exam papers, posed as specific questions (e.g. questions about issues relating to performer violence and drug use). You need to know examples, causes and possible solutions for all of these issues.

If the question asks you to 'discuss' a topic (e.g. 'Discuss reasons for and against the use of performance enhancing drugs in sport'), full marks can only be gained when both sides of the argument are given. In order to show your understanding of the debate surrounding various ethical issues in sport, you may have to make points you do not necessarily agree with (e.g. providing arguments in favour of the legalisation of drugs in sport). In addition, try not to dwell too long on a point you feel particularly strongly about, as purely repeating your arguments will limit the possible marks you can gain.

By the end of this topic, you should be able to:
- explain the terms 'amateurism' and 'professionalism'
- explain how elite sport is being professionalised and influenced by commercial forces
- give the effects, both positive and negative, of commercialism in sport, i.e. understand the ethics of sponsorship
- relate the Olympic Games to issues of commercialism

1 Definitions

- **amateurism:** participation in sport for the love of it rather than for extrinsic gain.
- **professionalism:** earning one's living from sport, where intrinsic values tend to be overshadowed by a full-time commitment to sport, with all the commercial connotations that it brings with it.
- **advertising:** promoting or making known to the public goods or services for sale.
- **sponsorship:** financial input into sport by a business or individual in return for advertising a company or product.

2 Commercialism

Elite sport is being professionalised and commercialised in a number of ways. The most obvious is the high financial rewards available for top performers in sports that receive media attention (e.g. golf, soccer and tennis). This may lead to an increase in the pressure to win, fostering a 'win at all costs' attitude and perhaps even cheating. Sport is sold as a product to the media (e.g. Premiership football or Super League rugby).

2.1 Sponsorship

Companies can become involved in sport in a number of different ways, including financing or sponsoring:
- a stadium, e.g. the Reebok stadium at Bolton
- a league/competition, e.g. the Guinness Premiership
- an individual, e.g. Nike sponsors Tiger Woods and Wayne Rooney
- a team, e.g. AIG was the principal sponsor of Manchester United for the 2007–08 season

2.1a Ethics of sponsorship

The involvement of sponsors in sport can be both positive and negative.

Reasons for sponsorship	Reasons against sponsorship
Sport is expensive to run and therefore requires a high level of financing.	Sponsors focus mainly on high-profile sports, teams, events or individuals.
The extra publicity may have a knock-on effect and ensure media coverage.	Sport may have to accept the intrusion of sponsors who may gain too much control over an event or sport and can dictate timing etc.
Increased revenue attracts top-level performers to an event or team.	Sponsorship can give an unhealthy image to sport (e.g. from gambling/alcohol companies).
Individual sponsorship allows full-time training.	Performance might suffer due to demands of the sponsor.

3 ## Case study: the Olympic Games

Following the bankruptcy of the Montreal Games in 1976, there was no public funding of the 1984 Los Angeles Olympics. Peter Uberoth led the LA Organising Committee along a commercial route to find the money, using strategies such as selling the Olympic logo and the television rights to the highest bidders. Every element of the Olympics had an official supplier.

The result was that all subsequent Games became dominated by private-sector funding, a pattern which looks set to continue. Cities now see huge benefits in hosting or bidding for the Games (for example London's successful bid for the 2012 Games). However, bidding has led to problems of corruption and bribery, for example the Salt Lake City scandal, when the organising committee was bribed.

Examiner's tip

Commercialism in sport is an important topic area for all the exam boards. You must be able to give examples of the different forms of sponsorship and demonstrate an awareness of the advantages and disadvantages of such sponsorship. Links between sponsorship, sport and the media (the 'golden triangle') should also be understood clearly and related appropriately to practical examples.

By the end of this topic, you should:
- know how the media can inform, educate and entertain the public
- be able to outline the media's role in advertising
- be able to suggest how the media might improve the involvement in sport of target groups

1 *Functions of the media*

1.1 Informing

The media tell the public what is happening in the world of sport. For example, newspapers, websites and television shows list the fixtures and results of many different sports. Popular sports, such as football, tennis and cricket, are reported on by the mainstream media; others are covered by specialist publications or websites.

1.2 Educating

The media are responsible for increasing public knowledge about sporting issues in the UK and around the world. For example, there are television documentaries on a range of subjects such as soccer hooliganism or drugs in sport. Programmes such as *Transworld Sport* (broadcast on Channel 4 and Sky Television) report on weekly events and topical issues in the sporting world. The BBC Sports Academy website is another excellent source of material designed to improve sporting knowledge.

1.3 Entertaining

A large amount of television and radio airtime and newspaper column inches is devoted to helping people enjoy their leisure time by either reading about, listening to or watching sport. Sport entertains and engages people, even when they are not participating in it directly. Examples of this include football World Cup matches, the World Athletics Championships, the Olympic Games and Twenty20 cricket.

1.4 Advertising

The media are important in helping to generate income for an individual, a team, a sport or an NGB by covering events or profiling individual performers. This attracts commercial interest from businesses. There are therefore strong and mutually beneficial links between the media and commercialism in sport.

The media and sponsors are attracted to sport because it has mass appeal, including the image of being 'cool' and 'trendy' to the young. This is evident in examples such as the use of Wayne Rooney in Nike football advertisements to promote sportswear, including lightweight football boots.

2 Women and the media

There are various ways in which the media can improve the involvement of women in sport. These include:

- increasing information about women's sport (e.g. providing results or coverage of women's football, rugby, cricket or netball)
- educating and entertaining through documentaries or newspaper articles publicising exciting female successes (e.g. Ellen McArthur, Michelle Wie)
- using female sports stars to advertise an activity and promote certain products (e.g. Paula Radcliffe is sponsored by Nike)

These principles can be applied to other target groups, such as ethnic minorities, people with disabilities and the elderly.

Examiner's tip

An understanding of the varied roles of the media, and their potentially positive effect on improving the involvement of certain target groups in sport, is required particularly by OCR Unit G451 and AQA Unit 3. It is important to be able to support your knowledge of sport and the media with practical examples.

TOPIC 10 Sport and culture

By the end of this topic, you should:
- be able to define the terms 'society' and 'culture'
- understand sport as a reflection of culture in Australia, the USA and the UK
- be able to explain how the Olympic Games are a vehicle for nation building
- know what ethnic sports are and be able to give their key features and reasons for survival in modern-day society

1 Definitions

- **society:** a community of people interacting with each other.
- **culture:** a product of society, often represented by that society's norms, attitudes and beliefs.

2 Sport as a reflection of culture

2.1 Australia

Native Australians (Aborigines) were presumed dangerous by European settlers and were forced to migrate inland by settlers who wanted their territory. Australia became a British colony at the end of the nineteenth century. Sports that were becoming popular in the UK, such as rugby and cricket, were exported to Australia, and many of these were adapted to the Australian style of play and developed their own identity, for example **Australian Rules football**. Today, Australians have a strong need-to-win ethic and place a high value on sport. Australia is a comparatively 'young' culture, seeking international identity, recognition and a chance to prove itself. There has been a high level of government investment in sport at all levels.

Australian Rules football has developed into a highly prominent game in Australia for several reasons:
- it is known as the 'people's game' and is accessible to all
- it reflects the 'frontier/manly' image of the bush in the aggressive way it is played
- it has an image of fair play, which suits Australia and its recognition for the 'best and fairest'
- it gives opportunities for commercialism through sponsorship and media coverage (games are played at strategic times throughout the week to attract the biggest audiences)

2.2 The USA

The USA is a world leader in many sports and supplies its sportsmen and women with excellent funding and facilities at all levels. The War of Independence (1863–66) severed links with Europe, and from this point US sport reflected the emergence of an American identity. Some sports were adapted from European sports, for example from rugby came 'gridiron', or **American football**; others were invented, for example James Naismith invented basketball in 1891.

The **American Dream** encapsulates the idea that everyone can achieve success through hard work, and sport is seen as a vehicle to rise up the social ladder. Another characteristic of the American attitude to sport is the '**win ethic**' — winning is the only thing that matters. This is also known as the **Lombardian philosophy**, named after Vince Lombardi, the head coach of the Green Bay Packers in 1959, who transformed them from a losing team into a major power in baseball.

The USA is a capitalist society based on private enterprise, in which commercialism is strong. Sport provides a focus for national identity — the 'stars and stripes', the oath and the national anthem all remind people of the nation's success, particularly when they are displayed and performed at global sporting events.

2.2a Education, PE and sport in the USA

- Education in the USA is predominantly free and provided by the state.
- Each state administers education through the local District School Board.
- PE is part of the curriculum — it is designed to improve the physical, mental, social and emotional development of the child.
- Sports are more important than PE in the USA. PE teachers have lower status and separate roles from sports coaches.
- Inter-school sport is important.
- Schools often have excellent facilities.
- The provision of sport in school can be elitist — resources are focused on the most able.
- Coaches are paid highly but are under pressure to produce results (e.g. in American football).
- Sports scholarships to universities are available — sport is seen by coaches as more important than academic studies.
- Sport provides entertainment and attracts commercial interests, even at high-school level.

2.2b Elite level sport in the USA

- The 'win ethic' is dominant; sport is used to prove the USA's status as a world superpower.
- Sport offers the promise of 'rags to riches' — everyone in society has a chance to be successful.
- Striving for excellence is developed through interschool/intercollegiate sport and sports scholarships.
- School sport generates its own funding, for example via media coverage.
- Commercial enterprises are involved with collegiate football and scholarships. Federal money is used to finance the Olympic team.

2.2c American football

American football emerged from the European game of rugby in 1879. It is now a highly paid professional sport in the USA. It has strong associations with:

- **violence** — it uses provocative language such as 'sack the opponent' and includes the wearing of protective body armour to reduce physical inhibition
- **commercialism** — the media desire for sensationalism and violence in American football sells sport to the public and means high financial rewards are available for top performers

American football teams have massive stadia to accommodate the large number of fans wanting to attend games. These fans are entertained in a family-oriented environment with lots of support entertainment alongside the actual game (e.g. cheerleaders).

2.3 UK

2.3a Ethnic sports

Ethnic sports are traditional events, particular to a certain social group, which have taken place for many years. Examples include mob football at Ashbourne and the Highland Games. They have many key features that can also be seen as reasons for their survival. For example, they:

- are usually annual
- are social/community gatherings
- help to maintain traditions and heritage
- attract tourists/are financially beneficial
- occur in rural or isolated areas

3 The Olympic Games and 'nation building'

China is a communist culture and, as with all areas of life, sport is under the authoritarian control of the government. Sport is used as an opportunity to endorse communism and to create a sense of national pride and collectivity. It also acts as a 'shop window' for a communist state to demonstrate its assets through sporting successes at global events.

The Olympic Games are often chosen as the stage on which communist states such as China try to prove their supremacy and show the world that their political system works best. High-profile and Olympic sports are chosen for investment by the state, with such funding often being disproportionately high in relation to other areas of society such as health and education. Economic benefits arising from hosting the Olympic Games in China may also be important for China's 'nation building', leading to increased tourism, media attention and investment in Chinese industry.

Examiner's tip

'Sport and culture' is a particularly important topic for OCR Unit G451. To help you remember the characteristics/reasons for survival of ethnic sports in the UK, you could use the acronym 'FISTA': F = financial; I = isolation; S = social; T = traditional; A = annual. AQA no longer requires an understanding of comparative issues in sport, but some of the features of sport in the USA are relevant when discussing sporting ethics in Unit 3.

By the end of this topic, you should be able to:
- describe the key characteristics of popular recreation activities
- describe the social setting/cultural factors within which the activities were found
- identify key characteristics of 'case study' activities such as mob football and pedestrianism in the era of popular recreation

1 *What was popular recreation?*

Popular recreation covers those activities and pastimes undertaken by the majority of the population before physical activity became 'rationalised' and divided into the sports we know today. Popular recreation activities were occasional and often linked to festivals that only happened a few times a year, for example mob football at Shrovetide. Such activities tended to be local, and certain areas devised their own version of an activity — a practice known as **local coding**. They were social occasions and reflected the agrarian and often isolated nature of the communities that took part in them. Betting on the outcome was popular.

Popular recreation activities were frequently violent and rowdy, involving animals and often resulting in damage to property. They provided an opportunity for the lower classes to let off steam, although the upper classes also took part in activities such as **real tennis**.

The number of participants in popular recreation was not limited and most activities, including mob football, were **not codified** (i.e. they had no rules). Low levels of literacy meant that any rules that did exist were not written down. Activities included blood sports, the cruelty of which reflected the harsh lives of the peasants. Physical force, rather than skill, was the key to success.

1.1 The social background to popular recreation
- Travel opportunities and communications were limited, so activities were restricted to the local vicinity.
- Society was feudal — the gentry owned the land; peasants worked for little return. Social classes were rigidly fixed. The two-tier society led to different pastimes for the upper and the working classes.
- Most people, especially the poor, were illiterate, leading to limited codification of activities.
- Hygiene and housing were poor. Sporting events were often a form of 'catharsis' — they provided relief from the harsh living conditions of society. Therefore, they were often violent.
- The majority of the nation's population lived in the countryside and therefore made use of natural resources in their recreation.
- Communities were small and everyone knew each other. Consequently, social occasions provided an opportunity for recreational activities.
- The peasantry worked long hours as dictated by the seasons and had little time for leisure, so their recreational activities were occasional. However, wealthy landowners had a large amount of leisure time and were able to enjoy recreational activities on a regular basis.

2 Classifying popular recreation activities

2.1 Game activities

- **Invasion games** included mob football, e.g. at Ashbourne.
- **Target games** included primitive versions of cricket, bowls, skittles and quoits.
- **Court games** — real tennis was an exclusive activity, as it required special facilities and equipment and had complex rules; poorer people played the game as 'rackets', without any specialist equipment.

2.2 Pedestrianism

Pedestrianism, also known as competitive walking, developed in the late sixteenth century. When travelling by coach, members of the gentry would send out footmen to make arrangements for when the party stopped for the night. Noblemen started to place bets on which footman would cover a certain distance in the shortest time. Footmen were chosen and trained for their athletic abilities. They were normally drawn from the lower classes, and their earnings from this activity were higher than from a normal job. Pedestrianism also offered excitement, including travel, and the prospect of earning money from prizes and wagers.

3 Development of sports and pastimes in river towns

Key words/reasons for the development of such activities:
- bathing — recreation — seasonal at bathing stations
- survival
- health/therapeutic/exercise for masses
- initial development of competitive swimming through the formation of clubs

Examiner's tip

OCR Unit G453 requires detailed knowledge of popular recreation. This section also covers information useful as a background for AQA Unit 3, which might require you to make comparisons between mob football and association football, for example.

Questions often focus on key characteristics of popular recreation activities and require examples to illustrate your knowledge. It is important to be able to relate these to the key features of the social scene in pre-industrial Britain, though given its harsh nature it is not always easy to do so. We now live in a highly technological world, which is reflected in the sports we play and how we play them.

You also need to be aware of why certain 'rural sports' and 'festivals' continue to survive in modern-day society (OCR Unit G451 links this to the continuing existence of 'ethnic sports' in the UK today). For OCR Unit G453, the historical studies option requires you to trace the development of a number of case study activities from the era of popular recreation through to modern-day society.

12 Public school influence on the development of sport

By the end of this topic, you should be able to:

- define the term 'public school'
- describe the characteristics of nineteenth-century public schools and their influence on the development of organised sport and games
- outline the development of sport and recreation in these schools
- recognise developments in women's education and their effects on sporting involvement
- describe the characteristics and development of public school athleticism and its influence on the development of rational sport and recreation in wider society

1 Public schools

A 'public' school is now called a 'private' school. Parents pay fees to have their children educated at these schools, which are often long-standing and sometimes accept children to board during term time. Public schools played a major part in the development and organisation of games and sports in the nineteenth century:

- As fee-paying/endowed schools, they could easily fund sports provisions and facilities.
- Boys in a boarding environment had lots of free time that needed occupying and energy that needed burning off.
- Pupils at such schools came from the upper classes. The gentry had experience of organising sports.

2 Popular recreation in public schools

2.1 Boy culture

The popular recreation activities carried out in public schools reflected the home lives of the boys who went there. Many sports and games were brought in from home and tailored to suit each school. They were adapted to suit the facilities the school had to offer, such as long corridors, quadrangles, courtyards or open grassy areas. This meant that there was a great variety of activities among schools. An example of this is the differences between mob football games depending on the school — Eton had the 'field' game, Rugby the 'handling' game and Harrow the 'dribbling' game. Public schoolboys had a large amount of free time to spend playing such games. Senior boys played the most active roles, with juniors collecting balls and so on. Gambling, drinking and rowdiness often surrounded popular recreation activities in pre-1800 public schools.

2.2 Dr Arnold and social control

Between 1820 and 1850, liberal headmasters such as Dr Thomas Arnold (headmaster of Rugby School) introduced reforms designed to produce responsible Christian gentlemen. The emphasis was on the concepts of godliness and manliness, and a broader curriculum was instituted so that boys had less time for idleness and mob games. Playground discipline was more rigorous, and was often under the control of a senior pupil. Games were seen as a means of social control through regular play — written rules, 'codes of honour' and a sense of loyalty to the school were established.

The expansion of games activities led to competitions both within and between schools, which were encouraged by headmasters keen to promote the successes of their schools. In turn, this led to the employment of specialist coaches and the provision of specialist facilities for sport. Such developments were influenced by the Clarendon Report (1864), which firmly placed team games as a way of developing character in public school boys.

2.3 The cult of athleticism

Athleticism is a devotion to sport that produces team spirit and group loyalty. It also develops manliness, self-discipline, physical endeavour, moral integrity and an appreciation of the value of healthy exercise.

Unlike the mid-nineteenth century, when boys engaged in gambling, drinking and fighting in their leisure time, the latter half of the century saw pupils' leisure time becoming a more 'civilised' opportunity for games, sports and competitions.

Sport was developed into a respectable, codified and well-organised aspect of public school education. Facilities such as playing fields were purpose-built. Games were played in a more 'ethical' manner, with a focus on responsibility, respect and morality. Links to **muscular Christianity** (i.e. a healthy mind in a healthy body to serve God) were developed — the aim was to win gracefully or lose with honour and bravery.

Physical endeavour and moral integrity became central features of sport in public schools. Ex-public school pupils took the cult of athleticism into society and encouraged working-class rational sport via the army, industry, church or indeed as returning teachers to their old public schools.

3 Public school influence on rational sport in wider society

The development of rational sport in public schools had a number of effects on society. Sport was promoted and developed further in all areas of the community by 'old boys':
- **The army** — as the British Empire grew, sport was taken all over the world, with all ranks of soldiers encouraged to play by army officers.
- **Industry** — industrialists/middle-class philanthropists began to see health benefits, improved attitudes and self-discipline as a result of sports participation for the workforce. Works teams and facilities were set up, and gradually more time was set aside for workers to play sports. The various Factory Acts eventually led to paid holidays for workers.
- **The Church** — the values of the Church were seen to be upheld in sport. This officially approved sport for all social classes. Churches developed teams for parishioners, and provided facilities for physical activity such as church halls. Sport was seen not only as a way of improving interest and attendance at church, but also as a means of social control, as it kept working-class males away from alcohol.

4 Women's education

Women's education was generally seen as unimportant in Victorian society, as women were viewed as inferior to men and only valued in the home. However, elite girls' schools and ladies' academies were developed in the late eighteenth century. They were for upper-class girls and taught the 'graces' it was felt important for women to have.

By the mid-nineteenth century, there was an emergence of girls' private schools (e.g. Roedean in Sussex). By the 1880s, tennis and cricket were being played in girls' schools, although the girls wore their normal clothing. Gradually, the perceived 'medical' reasons for women not participating in sport were set aside.

Examiner's tip

AQA Unit 3 and OCR Units G451 and G453 all require knowledge of the public school influence on the development of rational games. You need to be clear on the key changes made to sports by public schools during the late-nineteenth century and understand the links to athleticism and muscular Christianity during this period.

Always provide information relevant to the question set and to the period of time being examined. For example, if you are asked to give characteristics of public schools in 1800, you should focus on this specific period, rather than simply writing everything you know about sport in public schools in general. Questions are sometimes split into two parts, and you must address both parts in your answer. For example, 'Define the term "athleticism" and describe the underlying sports characteristics of public schools in 1870' requires two distinct answers. You should point out the values of the system, as well as outlining the 'rational' development of the games programme through factors such as rule development, regularity of play and support by teaching staff. Candidates often fail to do well in such questions.

You should ensure that when using a specialist term (e.g. athleticism or muscular Christianity), you illustrate your knowledge of what it means in precise terms.

OCR divides the public school development of sport into three distinct phases, which you need to be able to relate appropriately to the five case studies contained in the specification (i.e. bathing/swimming, athletics, football, cricket and tennis).

By the end of this topic, you should be able to:
- identify key features of rational recreation and compare it with a popular recreation activity (e.g. association football with mob football)
- outline the changes occurring in society and their impact on rational recreation
- state the key changes in the rationalisation of case study activities (e.g. bathing and swimming and track-and-field athletics)

1 Features

Rational recreation has several key features:
- It is rule-based (codified).
- National governing bodies are formed to control a sport.
- It is regular.
- It is respectable and governed by the idea of fair play.
- Referees and officials are present during play.

Rules for the conduct of a sport (e.g. scoring and the behaviour of the participants) were codified formally at all levels (for example, in football when the FA was established in 1863), from local through to international. This allowed competition on an agreed and equal basis. Public schools were important in the development of these rules, as they were needed for inter-school competitions. The gradual development of clubs, leagues and national governing bodies helped to develop and enforce rules nationally.

National and international competitions began to be held on a regular basis. This was aided by better transport, which led to greater access to sport for both spectators and participants. Professionalism increased as large numbers of people moved into towns and cities. Football clubs were built near town centres so that spectators and players could get to them easily.

2 Comparisons between popular and rational recreation

The table below shows the differences between mob football (popular recreation) and association football (rational recreation).

Mob football	Association football
No rules	Formal rules
No governing body	Governing body is the Football Association
No limits on number of participants, no time limits, no special kit	Number of players limited to 11 per team, time limit set at 90 minutes, each team has a recognisable and compulsory kit
Played irregularly, on festivals and holidays	Played regularly, e.g. on Saturday afternoons
Played on open rural areas	Played in a confined playing area
No organised competition	Leagues and national/international competitions
Little skill involved	High levels of skill required

3 Social class and sport

The gentry had an established full sports programme and plentiful leisure time. The emerging urban middle classes took these gentry sports and reorganised them according to amateur codes, which excluded financial rewards. The industrial working classes had little time for sport initially, but as the upper classes came to realise that sport was an important means of social conditioning, their leisure time increased. **Social Christians** and industrialists encouraged the development of organised sport for the workers, who were living in urban poverty.

3.1 Working hours and conditions

The development of the factory system at first gave workers little free time, with only Sunday designated as a day of rest. However, the Saturday half-day and the early closing movement gave workers time for organised sport. On seeing the health benefits and increased motivation sport could bring, some employers built sports facilities for their workers.

3.2 Urbanisation and leisure

The majority of the population of the country moved from rural areas to the cities. Groups such as the Church felt that these large concentrations of people needed meaningful leisure-time activities to divert them from drinking and gambling. This was catered for by:
- the building of public parks for walking and sports participation
- the provision of church halls
- the setting up of church teams in sports such as football

3.3 Communications and travel

- The improvement of the roads, the introduction of coach travel and the growth of the railway system meant that performers and spectators were able to travel around the country to attend sports events.
- Improvements in communications, such as the telegraph, meant that results and information could be sent quickly around the country.
- The development of newspapers meant that the wider public could keep in touch with the results of matches and events. As literacy increased, so did people's appetite for sports news.

3.4 The Church and sport

Major changes occurred in the Church's attitude to sport in the late-nineteenth century. A large number of church clubs arose out of **muscular Christianity**, which embraced ethical values such as team work, loyalty to a cause, conforming to rules, fair play and dedicating a performance to God. Ultimately, approval (and indeed encouragement) from the Church gave sport more status and value after industrialisation occurred.

4 Rationalisation of bathing and swimming

Bathing and swimming developed from leisure pursuits into organised activities and sports:

- Bathing stations were built initially on riverbanks, and spa towns developed with extensive bathing facilities.
- It became fashionable for the gentry to visit the seaside and participate in seaside bathing.
- The Wash-House Acts (1846) led to many industrial towns providing public baths for the working class.
- Swimming clubs were formed by members of the middle class; in 1874, the first National Championships were held, and the Amateur Swimming Association (ASA) was formed in 1884.

5 *The emergence of track-and-field athletics*

Modern-day track-and-field athletics developed out of professional walking and running. Pedestrianism was a form of walking race started by the gentry, who would place bets on which of their footmen could walk a certain distance in the shortest time. These footmen became professionals, competing against each other and against members of the gentry. Walking and running races over set distances were held either on racecourses or on open land.

Athletics was encouraged in public schools, as it adhered to the principles of muscular Christianity and physical endeavour. Schools ensured that the sport was organised and involved no wagering; it provided a social element to school life, as competitions could be held within and between schools.

The first governing body of athletics was the Amateur Athletics Club (AAC), set up in 1886. Pedestrians and professionals were not allowed to join or participate in events.

Examiner's tip

AQA, Edexcel and OCR all require a broad understanding of the development of rational recreation, including its key features and the main social influences during the time of the industrial revolution. Questions may also require a comparison with popular recreation.

You might be asked questions on the influence of specific organisations on the development of sport and recreation, such as the Church. Structured questions with a number of different parts may require knowledge of different topic areas, such as popular recreation, rational recreation and specific features of society as rational recreation emerged. Always look carefully at what the question is asking — you will not get marks for irrelevant information.

By the end of this topic, you should:
- know the key features of state PE before 1902
- know how state PE developed in the periods 1902–19 and 1919–33 (i.e. PT syllabus developments)
- be able to identify the key features of PE from 1950s *Moving and Growing* to National Curriculum PE (1988)

1 *Key features of state PE before 1902*

Before 1870, the education of those who could not afford to be taught privately was the responsibility of the Church. The majority, however, remained uneducated. The **Education Act 1870** was a first step towards a state education system. Most town schools had little space for playing fields or playgrounds, which restricted the sporting activities on offer.

Before the 1870 Education Act, physical education in schools was a mixture of Swedish, German and English gymnastics. Drill was introduced in the 1870s. It was taught by army non-commissioned officers (NCOs) and was for boys only. By the 1890s, some aspects of drill were being taught by teachers.

2 *Development of state PE, 1902–19*

State PE was influenced by the outcome of the **Boer War** (1899–1902), which saw the British Army defeated by a band of part-time soldiers. Many people blamed the defeat on the poor levels of health and fitness of the British Army, and this was seen as a consequence of poor physical training in schools. As a result, physical training remained an important part of the curriculum for decades.

2.1 1902 Model Course

The main features of the 1902 Model Course were that it was delivered by military instructors, and that fitness, familiarity with weapons and strict discipline were required. It was criticised for its strictness and lack of 'educational' objectives — the focus was on preparation for war (e.g. marching and using staves as weapons).

2.2 1904 Physical Training (PT) syllabus

This PT syllabus placed the emphasis on health and fitness. Specific lesson plans for teachers and instructors were drawn up, based on 109 exercise 'tables' and structured into three 20-minute lessons per week. The syllabus allowed for the poor facilities, large numbers of children and lack of equipment suffered by many schools.

2.3 1909 PT syllabus

This syllabus was more concerned with the welfare of working-class children, and had a slightly more 'therapeutic' angle. The number of exercise tables was cut to 71, and some organised games were introduced in their place.

3 *Further development of PT, 1919–33*

The First World War, during which a generation of young men was almost totally wiped out, had a profound effect on the education system. There was widespread recognition of the need for a more child-centred approach and the development of initiative within a disciplined environment. Women had taken on what were perceived as 'men's jobs' during the war, demonstrating that they could cope with physically demanding work and raising their social status. Thus women's education, including that in sport, began to be taken more seriously.

The 1919 syllabus allowed more freedom and individual interpretation in the use of the exercise tables, and time was set aside in each lesson for games and/or dancing. The 1933 syllabus allowed more game playing and group work and gave more choice to pupils and teachers. It was viewed as a 'watershed' between PT of the past and PE of the future.

4 *PE after the Second World War*

The **Butler Education Act 1944** placed the emphasis on equal access to education for all. Pupils experienced 'assault course' type equipment, including ropes, benches, ladders and climbing frames. They were required to use their own initiative and create activities for themselves. Modern dance and gymnastics were introduced too. The documents *Moving and Growing* (1952) and *Planning the Programme* (1954) were published by the Ministry of Education; these stressed the importance of variety, enjoyment and high levels of skill learning, and endorsed teaching in a more progressive/child-centred style.

5 *National Curriculum PE*

The **Education Reform Act 1988** led to the introduction of National Curriculum PE (NC PE). PE was made compulsory, thus reinforcing its position in the school curriculum. The aim is that pupils in schools should have similar experiences (i.e. uniformity) in PE, irrespective of where they live in the country. It applies to all state schools, although there may be variations in facilities, equipment and teaching, which may affect a pupil's PE experience.

NC PE is broken down into four stages:
- **Key Stage 1** is for children aged 5–7 years; it involves games, gymnastic activities and dance.
- **Key Stage 2** is for children aged 7–11; this involves six areas of activity: games, gymnastics, dance, athletic activities, outdoor and adventurous education, and swimming. Some choice is allowed for teachers in terms of the activities covered.
- **Key Stage 3** is for children aged 11–14 years; teachers have more choice in the areas of activity to focus on, with exercise activities introduced to NC PE from 2008.
- **Key Stage 4** is for children aged 14–16 years; a variety of activity areas are experienced from the curriculum options contained in the new programme of study for Key Stage 4, implemented in 2008. In addition to performing, there are also opportunities for officiating and coaching. Many schools include 'preparation for active leisure' in Key Stage 4 of their PE programmes, to try to reduce the 'post-

school gap'. By providing a breadth of attractive activities and linking to clubs and leisure centres, it is hoped fewer young people will drop out of sport/physical activity when it is no longer compulsory.

6 *Comparisons between military drill and PE in the 1950s*

Military drill	PE in the 1950s
No apparatus	Use of apparatus
Limited space	More space available
No choice	Individual choice of activity
Performed as individual	Group situations included
Regimented exercise	Play and freedom of movement allowed, skills developed, minor games played

Examiner's tip

Knowledge of the development of state education is required in AQA Unit 1 and OCR Unit G453. Many chief examiners' reports state that candidates suffer from 'poor exam technique' when responding to questions in this topic area. This is often caused by not devoting sufficient time and space to higher-mark questions and writing too much on lower-mark sections. Read the questions carefully and look at the marks allocated in order to avoid this pitfall. You must demonstrate clear and specific knowledge and not allow your answers to become too vague and generalised.